Index

Table of Contents

Foreword ....
    Foreword on the Goddard Method of *Judo* 6
    How to use the Goddard Method of *Judo* 7

Chapter 1 9
    Introduction 10

Chapter 2 11
    Strikes 12
        Principles and Patterns 12
        Basic Principle 12
        More Advanced Principles 13
        Key Principles for Strikes (Punches/Kicks) 14
            Timing of Kicks 15
            How to Better Execute Turning and Spinning Strikes/Kicks 15
            How to Progress from Turning Kick to Roundhouse Kick to Spinning Roundhouse Kick 16
            How to Apply Principle to do a Tornado Kick 18
        Damage and Power 18
            Damage 19
            Power 20
    Blocks 20
        Function of Blocks 22

Chapter 3 23
    Basic Principles You Need to Know for Throws and Groundwork 24
        How to Apply *Judo* 24
        How to Grip an Opponent 25
        Balance 26
        Stretch and Roll 28
        Generating Power for Throws 29
        Big Movement Versus Small Movements 30
        Movements for Throws 30
        Positions for Throws 30
        Three Throws to Use 31
        Key Points When Applying Throws 31

More Advanced Principles for Throws and Groundwork 32
Mental Discipline 32
Demonstrating Control 33

Chapter 4 35
Leg and Foot Throws 36
Core Technique – Leg Reap 36
Variations 36
How to Apply Core Technique – Minor Reap 37
Variations – Pin and Rotate 37
Variations – Foot Sweep 38
Core Technique – Heel Trip 38
How to Apply Core Technique 38
Variations 39
Core Technique – Propping Drawing/Wheeling 39
How to Apply Core Technique 39
Variations 40
Hand Techniques 41
Core Technique – Shoulder Wheel 41
How to Apply Core Technique 41
Variations 41
Core Technique – Body Drop 42
How to Apply Core Technique 42
Variations 42
Core Technique – Floating Drop 43
How to Apply Core Technique 43
Variations 43
Shoulder Throws 45
Core Technique 45
How to Apply Core Technique 45
Variations 45
Hip Techniques 47
Core Technique 47
How to Apply Core Technique 47
Variations 47
Sweeping Loin/Leg Techniques 50
Core Technique 50
How to Apply Core Technique 50

- Variations 51
- **Rear Techniques** 52
  - **Core Technique** 52
    - How to Apply Core Technique 52
    - Variations 53
- **Sacrifice Techniques** 55
  - **Core Technique – Circle Throw** 55
    - How to Apply Core Technique 55
    - Variations 56
  - **Core Technique – Drop Throws** 57
    - How to Apply Core Technique 57
  - **Core Technique – Side Rolling Throws** 58
    - How to Apply Core Technique 58
    - Variations 59

Chapter 5 61
- **Kata** 62
- **Modular Parts of Throws** 65
  - **Examples of Modular Throw Components** 66
    - Variation on a theme 66
    - Hybrid Principles 68

Chapter 6 72
- **Holding Techniques** 73
  - **How to Apply Core Technique** 73
    - Variations– "Chest Pin" Techniques 73
    - Variations – "Scarf Hold" Techniques 74
    - Variation – Kata-Gatame 75
  - **Moving Around the Body** 75
  - **Modular Parts of Holding Techniques** 77
- **Limb Locking Techniques** 78
  - **General Principle** 78
    - Variations 78
- **Strangling Techniques** 81
  - **General Principle** 81
    - Variations - Chokes 81
    - Variations - Strangles 82

- **Postface** 85
  - *Judo* **Technique List** 86

Throwing Techniques 86
Ashi-waza - Foot and Leg Techniques 86
Koshi-waza - Hip Techniques 86
Te-waza - Hand Techniques 87
Sutemi-waza - Sacrifice Techniques 87
Groundwork Techniques 88
Kansetsu-waza - Limb Lock Techniques 88
Osae-komi-waza - Holding Techniques 88
Shime-waza - Strangling Techniques 88
Glossary of Terms 89
Dedication 90
Acknowledgements 91

Foreword

Introducing the Goddard Method of *Judo*

Foreword on the Goddard Method of *Judo*

Some key themes and principles running through this book

People can become overwhelmed with the level of detail in lessons, books and YouTube videos. My book aims to be the key that unlocks your understanding and potential so you can get the most out of lessons and YouTube presentations etc. I have included instructions that break down techniques into bite-size chunks to help you better understand what you are doing when taking lessons, looking at reference guides, or perhaps learning new moves with a partner.

How to apply *judo* moves is standard practice; my book is about how to interpret this standard practice.

I have deliberately picked similar description styles on how to execute the moves, to show patterns and links. Other books concentrate on the technical side of *judo*, whereas my book emphasises the pattern/spirit in easy-to-remember key points. It also includes technical information on how to improve your *judo* as you gain experience.

There are many and varied *judo* techniques which can be performed in a variety of positions. There are too many variables for me to mention all of them in this book, so I have focused on a quick-start guide to techniques. Once you have tried them in the order I have suggested, you can fit them together in different combinations.

The box below is what a Goddard tip looks like – where you see one, it is one of my key things to remember, to help you improve your *judo*.

> (Example Text).

How to use the Goddard Method of *Judo*

Chapters 1, 2 and 3: What you see is what you get. These can be read as independent chapters.

Chapter 4: Using *hip techniques* as an example.

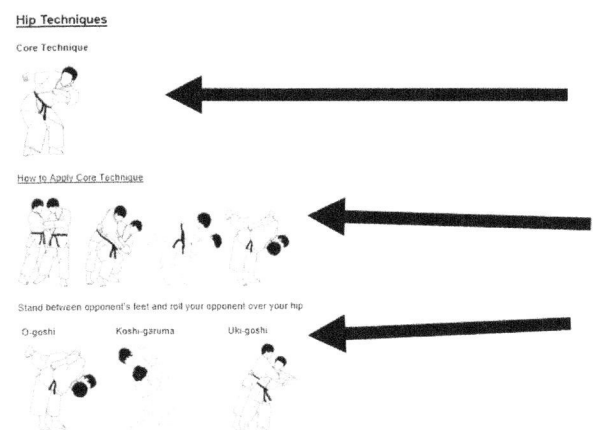

Stand in the core position

Use this kind of entering technique

Change how you grip an opponent, and where you stand, as per the variation illustrations to get multiple uses out of one movement

Chapter 5: Builds on Chapter 4 to show how parts of different throws can be combined to make other techniques. For example:

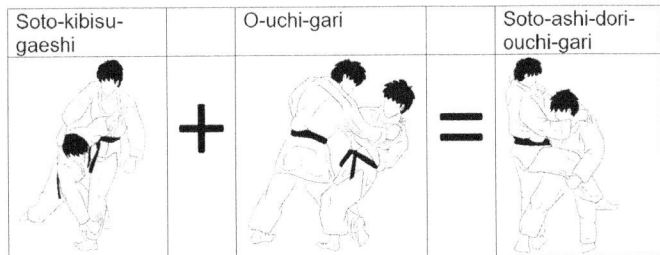

Chapter 6: Shows how principles for throws in Chapter 4 (use core movement in different positions) can be applied in groundwork.

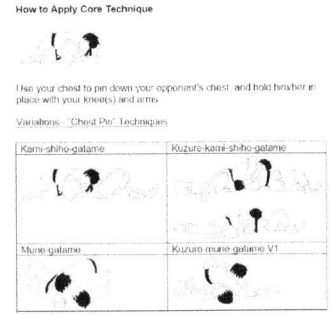

Chapter 1

Introducing the Goddard Method of *Judo*

Introduction

The martial art of *judo* developed from *ju jitsu*. It originally included techniques people would recognise today in *Brazilian ju jitsu* (throwing and grappling), *shotokan karate* (blocks and strikes), and *aikido* (some weapons techniques).

Techniques have been added and removed from the judo syllabus over time. There is now more focus on throwing, joint locks and strangles/chokes. Blocks, strikes, weapons techniques and *kata* (a series of pre-arranged moves) are infrequently taught in modern *judo*.

As competition rules change, some older techniques can no longer be used, and so have dropped out of favour. They can be used in *randori* (free practice), but *judokas (judo* practitioners) tend to focus on techniques that can be used in competition.

My book will introduce you to the principles behind throws, holds, chokes/strangles, blocks and strikes. These are for techniques from old and new syllabuses. You'll be able to see how a few key principles can unlock many techniques

Chapter 2

Strikes and Blocks

Although strikes and blocks are not used in competition, they are still practised in *judo katas*, so knowledge of these are still required to cover all the elements of *judo*.

Strikes

Principles and Patterns

There are key principles and patterns that make techniques work. If you focus on these rather than individual techniques, you will be able to learn more, faster.

Parts of the body to strike with:

Arm	Hand	Leg	Foot
• Elbow.	• Palm heel. • Knuckles of index and middle fingers (punches). • Edge of hand from the little finger to the wrist (knife hand and hammer fist strikes).	• Knee. • Shin (kicks).	• Ball or heel (kicks).

Basic Principle

> Basic principle: Aim   >   Strike   >   Retract.

Example strikes: *Cross punch* and *front kick*.

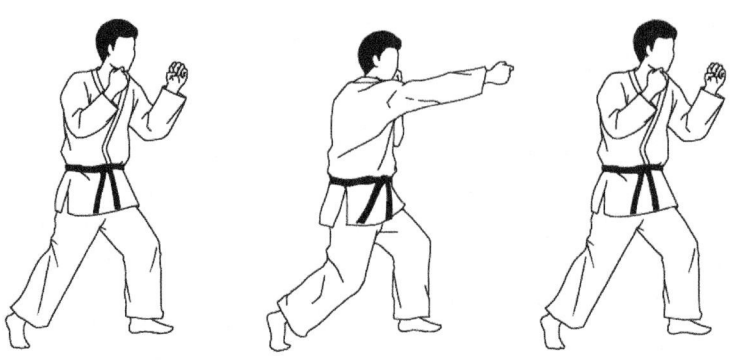

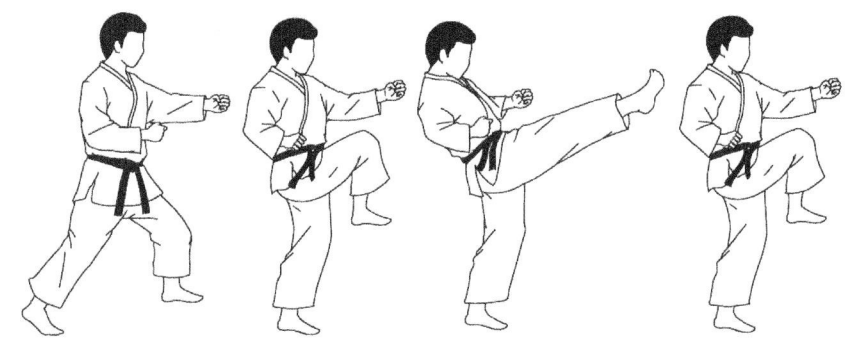

More Advanced Principles

You can add more components to make techniques more complicated.

| Aim > Jump > Strike > Retract. |

Example strikes: *Jumping front kick* and *jumping front scissor kick*.

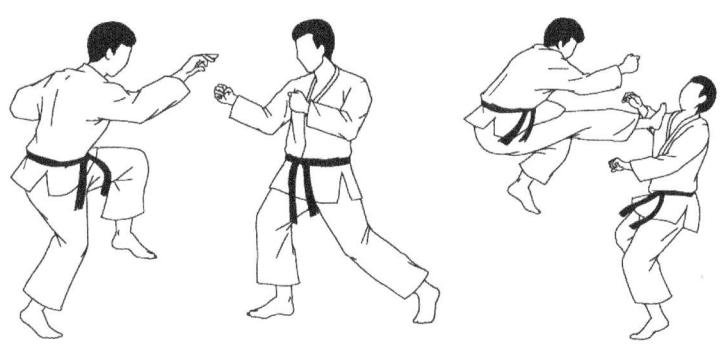

| Aim > Spin > Strike > Retract. |

Example strikes: *Spinning hammer fist, back turning kick* and *roundhouse kick*.

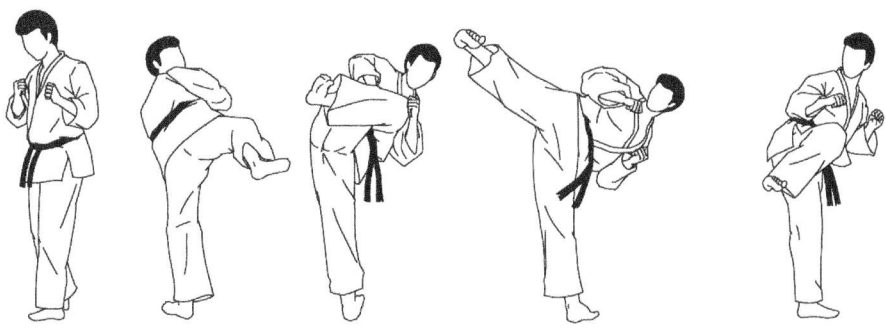

| Key principle to execute technique: Turn > Turn > Recover. |

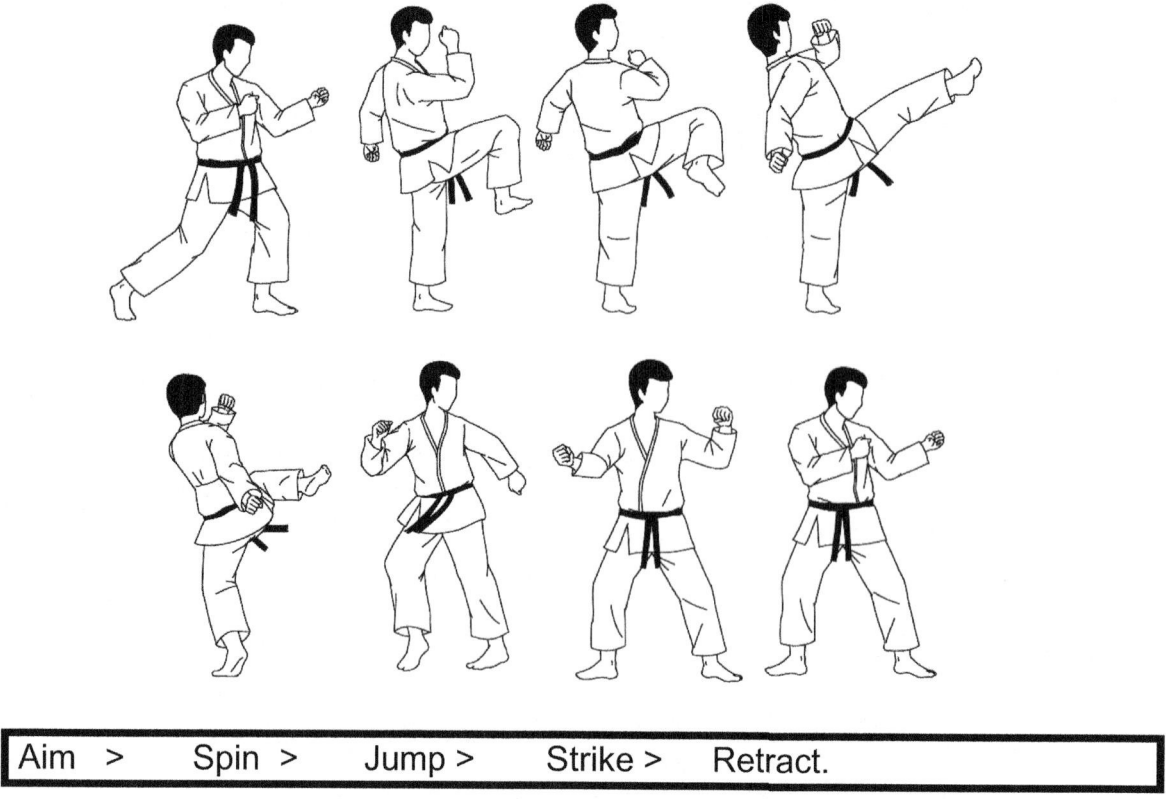

Aim > Spin > Jump > Strike > Retract.

Example strikes: *Jumping back kick* and *jumping spinning side kick*.

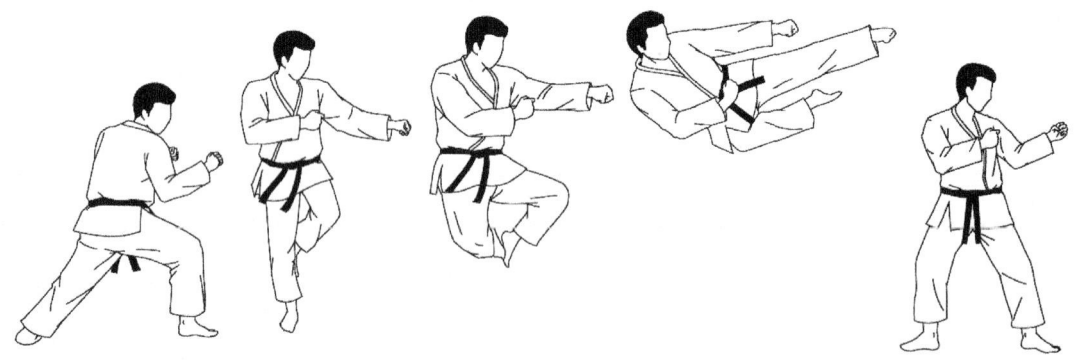

These principles/techniques work the same way in other martial arts such as *tae kwon do.* In case you wish to use what you know in *judo* to help you learn a new martial art faster. Or if you have to apply what you know against another martial art in mixed martial art competition.

Key Principles for Strikes (Punches/Kicks)

Aiming tip for kicks and punches:
- Where your shoulders point is where the strike is aimed.
    - Front strikes: Face forward.

- o Side strikes: Where deltoid/shoulder joint points.
- o Turning strikes: Take shoulder past target.
- The same principles apply to all arm and leg strikes, not just kicks and punches.

Timing of Kicks

You should be able to execute a straight kick e.g. a *front kick* in the time it takes you to say 'ver-dum' or '1, 2'.

You should be able to execute (Aim > Turn > Strike > Retract) a sideways or turning kick e.g. a *hook kick* in the time it takes you to say 'ver-der-dum' or '1, 2, 3'.

How to Better Execute Turning and Spinning Strikes/Kicks

Expand/contract in the shape of a tear drop. Turn your body half/full circle in the round end and extend your leg in the (narrow) 'tail'.

For example, *spinning back kick*: Expand by extending leg. Contract to spin on spot.

Step 1	Step 2	Step 3	Step 4

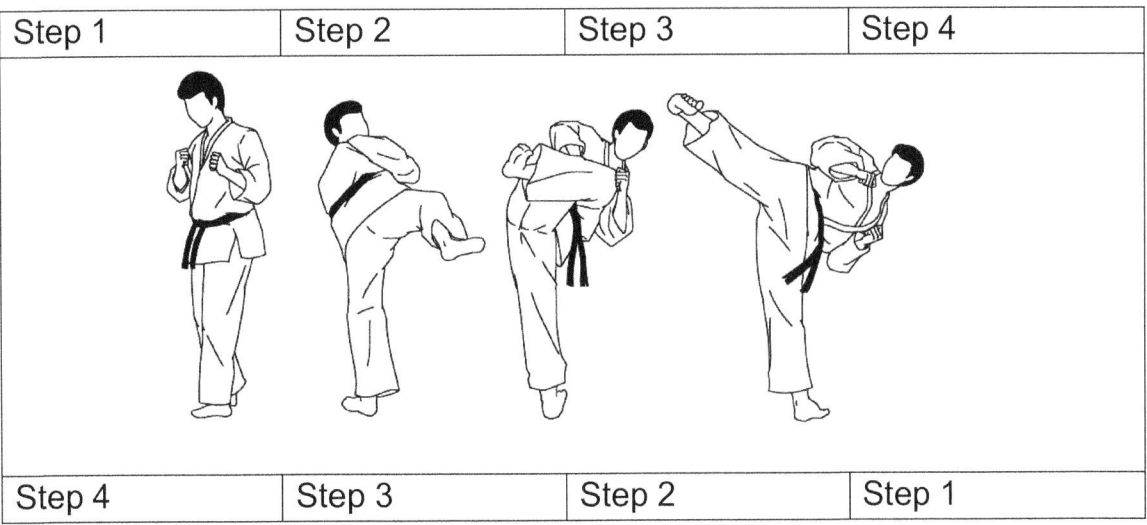

Step 4	Step 3	Step 2	Step 1

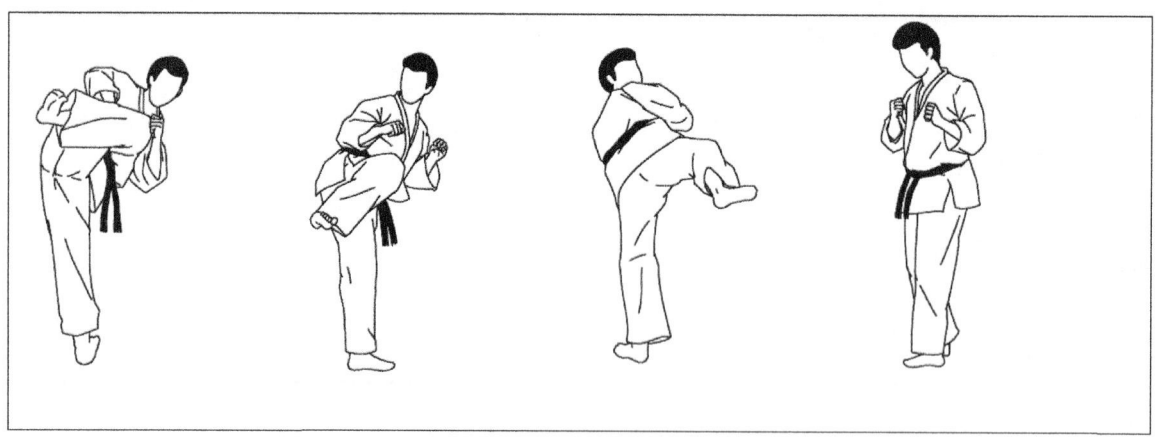

If you do 1, 2, 3, 4 to extend your leg; you should do 4, 3, 2, 1 to retract from the strike.
- Follow all stages in the process: Aim > Turn > Strike > Retract > Turn > Replace foot on floor (four stages to extend leg and four stages to retract it).
- A common error is to start by turning body then lifting the leg, then finish by turning body then planting leg; instead of planting your leg then turning your body (to settle balance).

> Key principle that applies to all striking techniques: Whatever you do to extend a limb to strike, do exactly the same in reverse order to retract (can be in different directions though e.g. 180 degree movement arc [*turning kick*] or 360 degree [*spinning back kick*]).

More principles:
- Keep foot near hip when kicking.
  Stepping and turning automatically cocks limbs e.g. spinning back kick.
- Strikes:
  - Draw limb across body in a tight arc to hide movement. Also to get expand/contract effect.
  - One-off technique: Turn > Turn > Recover.
  - Combination of techniques: Even number of 'turns'; 2, 4, 6, 8 etc then 'recover to finish e.g. Turn > Turn > Turn > Turn > Recover.
    - 'Recover' is like a full stop at the end of a sentence. It brings things to a halt.

How to Progress from Turning Kick to Roundhouse Kick to Spinning Roundhouse Kick

Use techniques you learnt in judo to understand the mechanics of other martial art techniques.

Use tools in Goddard Method of Judo ('what', 'how', 'when' and 'ready reckoners') to understand how to do new techniques faster.

Turning Kick

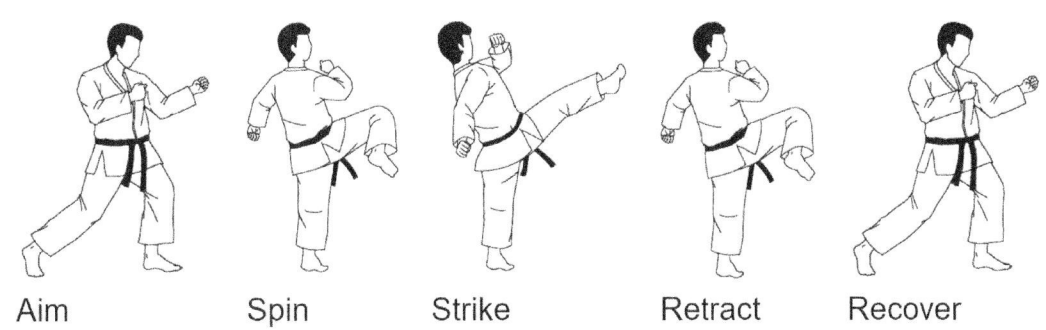

Aim   Spin   Strike   Retract   Recover

Roundhouse Kick

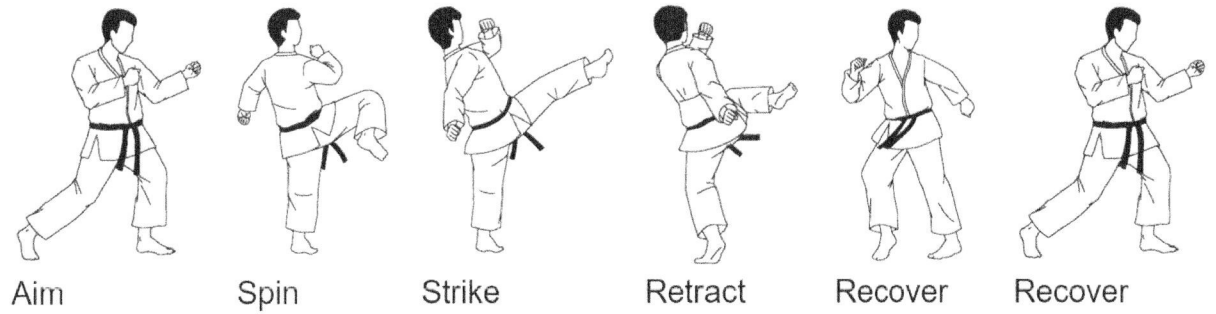

Aim   Spin   Strike   Retract   Recover   Recover

Spinning Roundhouse Kick

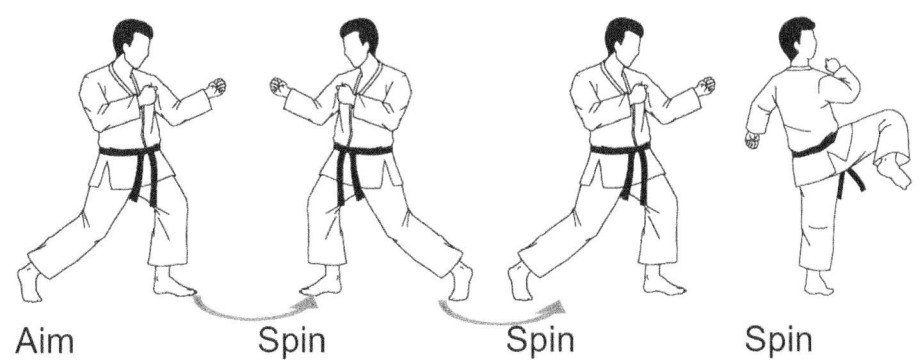

Aim   Spin   Spin   Spin

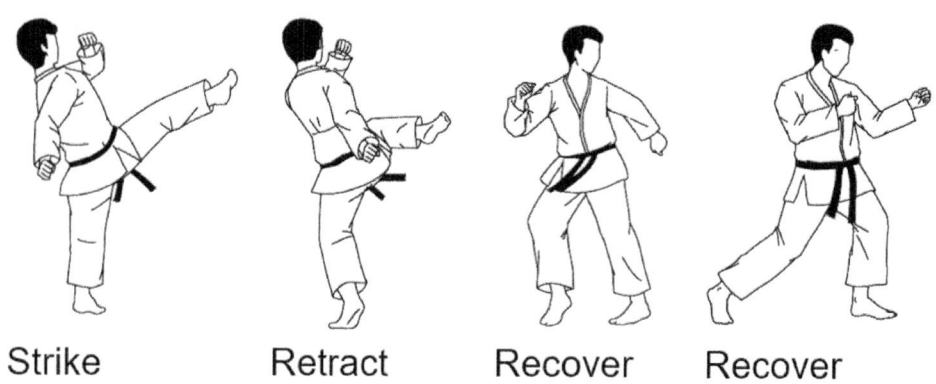

Strike   Retract   Recover   Recover

Front and rear legs change places along the same axis. This is hard to see when person demonstrating is not standing on a line. Placement of feet can limit arc of spin. The person doing the kick needs to complete a 360 degree turn to build momentum then another 360 degree turn to deliver the kick.

How to Apply Principle to do a Tornado Kick

If you are interested in trying *tae kwon jumping spinning kicks*... remember my principle of Aim > Spin > Jump > Strike > Retract. I have noticed kickers move in an ellipse not a circle. Move more like pivots (see Goddard Method of Ballroom and Latin Dancing book chapter 6)....straight forward then a fast 180 degree turn (repeat) then strike. That's how tornado kick etc. work.

Front and rear legs change places along the same axis. This is hard to see when person demonstrating is not standing on a line. Therefore it helps if you know what to look for in books, videos and demonstrations. Placement of feet can limit the arc of your spin. The person doing the kick needs to complete a 180 degree turn to build momentum then another 360 degree turn to deliver the kick.

Damage and Power

Martial arts are often taught or branded as sports in modern society. They began as fighting arts to train to defend yourself and fight off attackers, if not take the offensive(!). As such the point of training was to increase the ability to generate powerful strikes to damage (i.e. injure or kill) opponents.

The 'fighting art' side of martial arts continues to be taught to be armed/uniformed services.

People can learn martial arts for self-defence; but the focus in modern martial arts is to demonstrate power/control in civilised ways such as breaking boards, scoring points or knocking out an opponent (not permanently damaging them) in sparring/competition.

Damage

In order to cause maximum damage, there must be a balance between the three elements of power, framework and stability.

Take away any one of the above and the pyramid (i.e. amount of damage caused) shrinks. For example, it is not possible to deliver a powerful strike if your framework is poor (i.e. you are off-balance). Energy will be siphoned off from the blow as your body tries to stay upright. Your strike will also be easier to intercept/counter by your opponent.

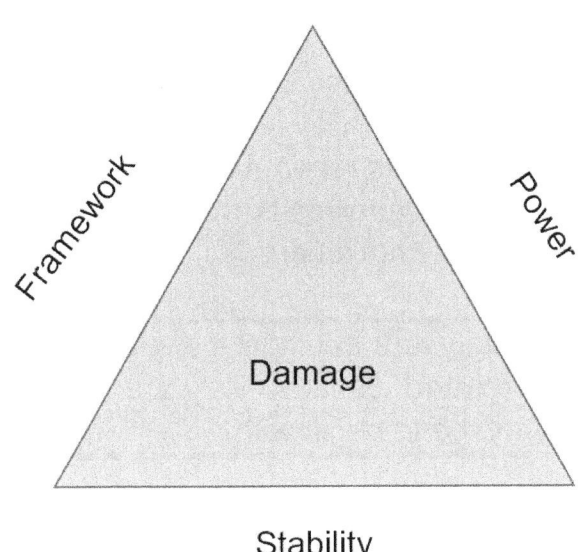

Key:
- Framework – how you stand.
- Power – the amount of force you put into a strike.
- Stability – you need to be on balance when delivering a strike.

Power

> Power = Mass x Velocity.

Over time, speed becomes more important than strength or muscle mass. You can develop more power faster through improving your speed/technique than by building extra muscle mass. Potential muscle mass is limited by your body size and ability to exercise. Whereas, the more you practise, the more energy efficient, faster and more accurate your techniques become; so power is not limited purely by your body size.

As detailed in *Key Points When Applying Throws - Basic Introductory Principles for Throws and Groundwork*: 'Power' for strikes can be generated by using your opponent's speed and direction against them (i.e. countering their movements). So this principle has several applications.

Similarly, as detailed in *Key Points When Applying Throws – Generating Power for Throws*: 'Power' for strikes develops from your stance foot position through to hip rotation and upper body movement.

> Note: An unfortunate reality is that bigger people find it easier to generate power than smaller people do, because they are naturally stronger and so have a significant advantage to begin with.

The aim of *judo* is for you to learn how to use your abilities and techniques in the most efficient way.

Blocks

> Basic principle: Aim   >   Block   >   Retract.

Examples of common blocks:

Rising	Lower

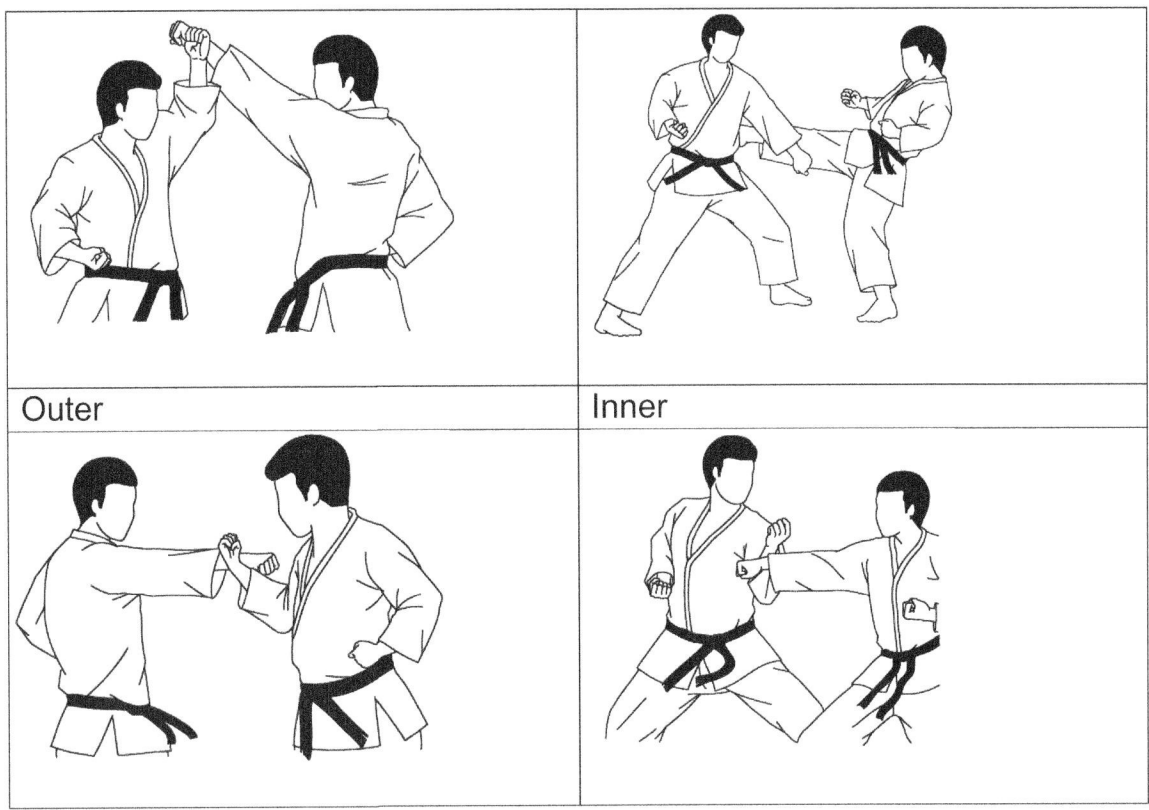

Use the outer or inner forearm to block strikes to begin with. These are strong areas of the body and large surface areas to make contact with (i.e. more likely to work for the inexperienced martial artist).

You can use other parts of the body such as hands as you gain more experience. This is a smaller surface area to try and hit an attacking limb with, but the power can be focused into a smaller area, making it more effective.

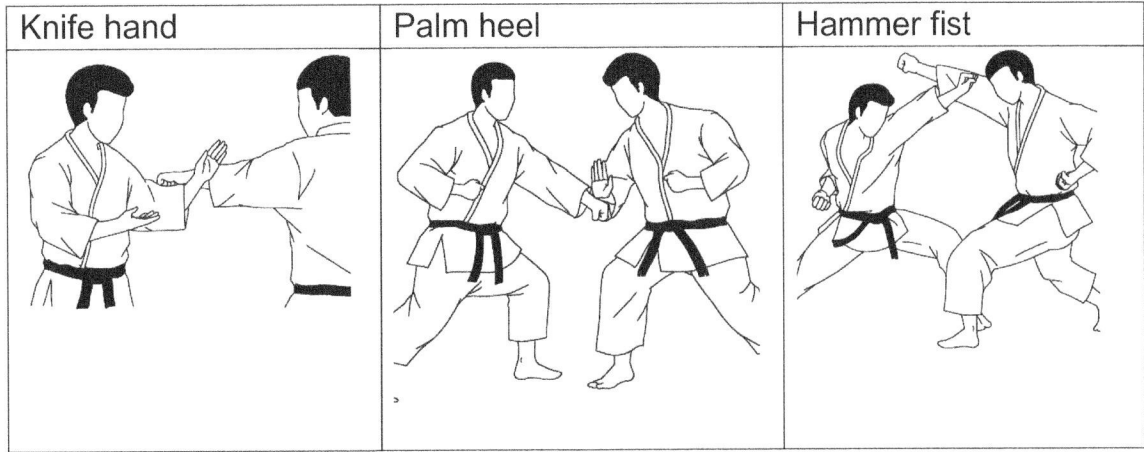

Function of Blocks

There are three ways that blocks can be applied:
- Defensively e.g. *elbow up block* or *knee up block* as used in *Thai boxing*. You take the impact of your opponent's strike on your limb by using it as a shield.
- As a parry to redirect your opponent's strike.
- Offensively e.g. *elbow down block* or *knife hand block* to strike your opponent's striking limb. In advanced forms of this technique, you can combine a block and strike to opponent's body at the same time. For example, if your opponent launches a *'haymaker' hook punch* to your jaw, you could retaliate with a *'short'* (i.e. more compact) *hook punch* to your opponent's jaw. Your punching arm will launch your strike and block your opponent's strike at the same time.

Chapter 3

Principles for Throws and Groundwork

- Basic Principles
- Advanced Principles

In this chapter you will find a series of principles on how to apply *judo*. This is information you need to know: not necessarily 'basic' or 'advanced', just how to apply *judo*.

Basic Principles You Need to Know for Throws and Groundwork

The following sections set out some basic principles to help you understand how techniques work. Later chapters in the book give you more details on which you can focus to help you get more out of lessons and YouTube videos. That is, to really understand how techniques work; so that you can learn, adapt and re-use principles in different ways and combinations.

Something that I noticed not being emphasised enough by some teachers is that it feels different when applying *judo* on different people. Everyone has a different body build, moves in different ways; they even (frequently) change stances when applying *judo*. You can attempt the same technique on different people and it will feel different each time, necessitating subtle changes in how to apply the technique each time. Explaining all of these variations is too complicated for a book or short video demonstration; you need to attend a class and practice on real people.

Judo has many techniques, so you can choose the 'right tool for the job'. That is, which one is the most appropriate for you to apply on the opponent in front of you.

How to Apply *Judo*

Below are my thoughts on the key principles to remember with techniques. Treat these as a skeleton to hang further details on. I suggest learning these first, try some techniques, learn through play (practice, practice, practice!) then add detailed knowledge as you gain experience.

Grip >   Wrap   >   Throw
Grip >   Wrap   >   Lock
Grip >   Wrap   >   Strangle
Grip >   Wrap   >   Hold down

Note; 'Wrap' means hold onto your opponent and then wrap:
- Them around your body. (For throws.)

OR

- Your limbs around your opponent. (For locks, strangles and hold downs.)

See *How to Grip an Opponent* below.

| What   >   How >   When |

Some people focus just on 'what' to do. By also learning 'how' and 'when' you will be able to progress by combining moves together in different ways.

| Like serving a portion of chips in a takeaway: Scoop > Wrap > Serve. |

The correct actions need to be performed in the correct order or the process will not work. For example, there is no point serving a bag that is empty, because no chips have been scooped first.

Likewise, you cannot wrap then throw someone if you do not grip them correctly first.

| The secret of *judo*: Grip > Wrap > (Technique) e.g. throw, lock or hold. |

This is the basic principle, but there are many subtleties in how to apply principles so you can perform techniques on an opponent. For example:
- Height.
- Strength.
- Weight.
- Reach (of limbs, specifically arms).
- Balance (specifically which foot is forward as this will influences someone's centre of balance).
- Determination.

The above factors will influence what techniques *judokas* will choose to perform on each other. For example:
- A tall *judoka* may prefer to use a leg reap technique (e.g. *o-soto-gari*) on a shorter *judoka*.
- A short *judoka* may prefer to use a shoulder throw technique (e.g. *morote-seoi-nage*) on a taller *judoka*.

How to Grip an Opponent

Variations on grips that can be used:
- Sleeves/arms of jacket.
- Lapels.

- Around waist, including holding the belt.
- Around shoulders.
- Legs of *judogi* (in *randori* (free practice) but no longer allowed in competition).

Balance

The choice/opportunity for a throw depends on the location of your balance and your opponent's. You will have to disrupt/break your opponent's balance in order to throw or roll them over.

You can either try and create an opportunity by provoking or tempting your opponent into making a move, or be more defensive and react to the actions of your opponent. Generally, you will do a little of both when practising.

Your balance is usually aligned forty-five or ninety degrees to the direction that your feet face. For example, your feet face forward in *front stance*, so you are vulnerable to diagonal attacks. If someone attacks your 'front' whilst you are in side stance, they may choose to use a sacrifice technique such as *tomoe-nage* that lets them drop between your spread feet and so turn the stability of your stance against you.

Strengths and weaknesses in stances listed below assumes that your opponent is standing facing you as per the arrows. Arrows show the direction in which a stance is strong. Solid black lines under the figure show directions of weakness. The dotted disc is the floor the figure is standing on.

Front stance	Side stance	Back stance
Traditional	Traditional	Traditional
Modern	Modern	Modern
Weight is mostly on front leg.	Weight is evenly spread over both legs.	Weight is mostly on rear leg.

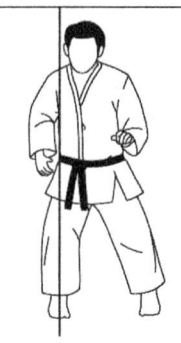	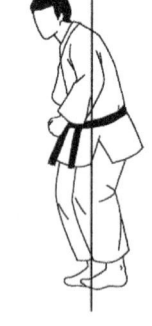	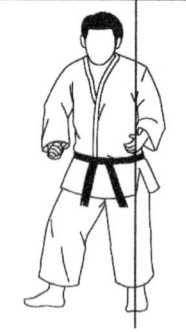
This is a versatile stance from which you can perform most strikes, blocks and throws.

The stance provides strong resistance from the front, but is weak against attacks from the forward and rear diagonals.

The rear leg provides a strong root for balance, but can be reaped by techniques such as *o-soto-gari* or *o-soto-gake*. | Provides strong sideways attack/defence potential. Weak from the front or rear (including diagonals).

The lower you go by spreading your feet, the less mobile you may become. It may be better to sacrifice a little framework strength by using a higher posture to gain speed of movement.

The stance has high sideways mobility to deliver sideways attacks (*side kick, o-uchi-gari etc.*), but your back two limbs are out of reach so can only play a limited role. | Can be used offensively or defensively.

Can be used in grappling situations as the basis for sweeps and throws.

The rear leg provides a strong root for balance, which may hinder mobility. |

Stretch and Roll

Judo throwing and groundwork rolling techniques follow manual handling principles.

Details below can apply to *judo* (standing) throwing and groundwork rolling techniques, but mainly apply to throws.

> You have to move your opponent on two separate axes (think of a globe) to break their balance.

Your opponent's shoulders give an indication of their balance and which way to rotate them to break their balance.

To break someone's balance:
- First break opponent's vertical alignment of head, hips and feet; usually by lifting/rolling them.
    - When I say "lift", I **DO NOT** mean heave them over using brute force. (See below.)
    - Clasp hold of opponent and move your body in the direction you want your opponent to go. This brings them with you.
    - Once your opponent's heels are (lifted) off the ground, they are vulnerable to being thrown. Getting your opponent to 'stand on tip-toe' is fine, you do not need to completely clear their feet off the floor, but it is very hard to throw someone when they are flat footed as this is when they are braced/balanced.
- Second, throw opponent off balance by rotating (around) horizontally, then follow up with a strangle or hold down if possible.

For example, *o-goshi* hip throw. Grip opponent > Wrap them into you > Continue movement to roll them across your hips (lift opponent onto toes to break balance) > Continue rotation movement to throw them off your back.

Generating Power for Throws

As per manual handling principles, push from your legs to get strength/power then transfer energy: Legs > Hips > Shoulders.

Turn your shoulders to get movement, like using a steering wheel in a car.

> Turn your shoulders by thrusting forward lead shoulder and winding back rear shoulder.

It is especially important to remember this point: When someone is in front of you, the natural subconscious reaction is to assume there is an obstruction, and so not move the front shoulder (closest to opponent), but try and move the rear shoulder. At best this reduces the power of your technique as it slows the rotation speed and diminishes its movement. At worst, it totally sabotages the technique and stops it working. Many *judokas* can't throw another *judoka* as they are too polite to barge through another's personal space.

Big Movement Versus Small Movements

Some throws use big movements and some use small movements. This will alert you in advance what you should be doing, therefore a:
- 'Small movement' throw will be telegraphed to an opponent if a 'big movement' is used.
- 'Big movement' throw will not work if a 'small movement' is used. (Not enough movement of power.)

For example:

Big movement	Small movement
O-soto-gari	Ko-soto-gari
O-goshi	Uki-goshi

Movements for Throws

> Movements for throws: Shoulder > Hip > Shoulder.

Perform an action such as a kick/throw like driving a car. Turn shoulder/steering wheel for direction > Move hip/press accelerator to get power. You need to use the correct mix of power and direction.

Direction	Power
Shoulder (person)	Hip (person)
Steering wheel (car)	Accelerator (car)

For example, when turning to apply *o-soto-gake* as a counter to *tai-otoshi*: You need to perform a five part process (move shoulder > hip > shoulder > hip > shoulder) to make a complete turn in order to get yourself in the correct position to counter opponent's technique. Most people only do two parts (shoulder > hip) so their foot/leg (and therefore all of them i.e. whole body) is in the wrong place.

Positions for Throws

Once a principle has been learnt, it can be applied in up to six ways/positions:
- Front.
- Left or right side (of opponent).
- Inside or outside of opponent's legs.
- Behind.

- Kneeling.
- Dropping.

By concentrating on principle(s) it is possible to use the same technique in some or all of the six different ways/positions. For example, *harai-goshi* is a hip throw with a leg sweep. Applications:
- Front: *O-guruma*.
- When standing outside of opponent's legs: *Uchi-mata*.
- When standing inside of opponent's legs: *Harai-goshi*.

Other martial arts may add 'jumping' as a seventh position, but this is rarely used in *judo* (such as a method of quickly closing the gap with an opponent e.g. jumping into a throw such as *kani-basami*), so I have only specifically referred to jumping in Chapter 2 *jumping kicks*.

Throws are made up of modular parts: Arms, bodies and legs. I will cover this in more detail later in the book (see Chapter 5).

Three Throws to Use

It seems to me that if you learn *o-soto-gari*, *ippon-seoi-*nage and *o-goshi* then you have three key throws to cover all sizes or opponent. So, you should have options for dealing with someone the same size, bigger or smaller than yourself.

If you then think of throws as made up of three parts (arms, legs and body); you can mix these up as required to give yourself more options. For example, I would say *sode-tsuri-komi-goshi* is the body and leg part of *o-goshi* with different arm grips.

Key Points When Applying Throws

Key principles to remember when applying throws:

- When the way is open, go forward (attack if your opponent is vulnerable).
- When the way is blocked, go around. (If the technique doesn't work, change direction.)
- Pull when opponent pushes, push when opponent pulls.
- Turn opponent's strengths into weaknesses, turn your own weaknesses into strengths. For example, make stronger opponents over commit

power/speed (potential strength) by using yielding skill (own lack of power potential weakness). This is a way to break an opponent's balance.
- Invariably single attacks do not work:
    - Try combinations of techniques.
    - Try applying the same technique two or three times in succession. If this does not work, try another technique. You have to balance persistence/commitment with not being predictable and so open to counters.
- The simplest way to counter a technique is to apply what your opponent is trying on you back on them. For example, swallow counter: Apply *o-soto-gaeshi* (a variation of *o-soto-gari*) on an opponent who is attacking with *o-soto-gari*.

More Advanced Principles for Throws and Groundwork

Mental Discipline

Belief/commitment is key to making techniques work. Think of Luke Skywalker failing to lift the X-Wing fighter out of the swamp in the *Empire Strikes Back* film because he did not believe he could do it (using the Force).

Take away any one of the above and the pyramid collapses (i.e. technique fails).

The body does what the brain tells it. If you have a clear idea in mind of what you want to do, and commit to doing it, the technique will work. If not, the body has no instructions to follow and so it does not work.

Instead of saying "I cannot do this", try a starting point of "I do not know how to do this, but I shall find out and then practise until I can do this".

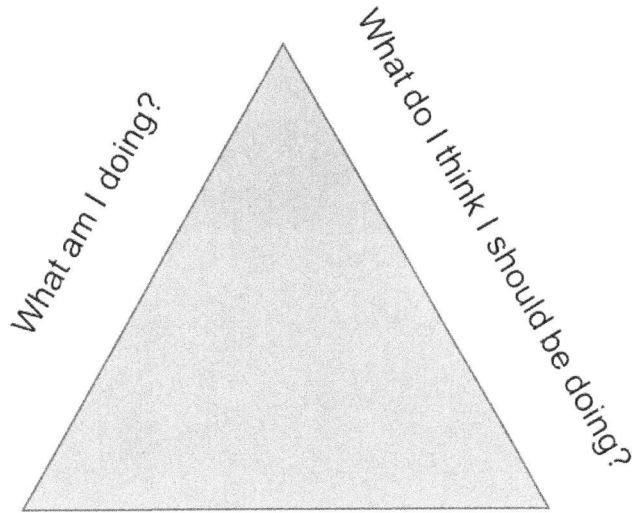

What should I actually be doing?

Demonstrating Control

To demonstrate full control of your opponent when throwing them:
- Apply a 'waterfall' movement: Take your opponent across your body then down to the floor, it will look like water going over a fall to an observer.
- Complete the movement. Don't let go of your opponent near ground. Instead, throw them to the mat, pin them there, then apply a ground hold etc. if possible.
- Pin opponent on their back.

> Never commit to one technique so much that you cannot follow up with a second one. Try and position yourself so that it is possible to flow from one technique to another to give you options in case a technique fails (perhaps your opponent moves or applies a counter technique). This will allow you to proceed from one technique to another in a series of combinations until you succeed.

The 'waterfall' movement is best exemplified by *sumi-otoshi*. If the technique does not work, you can apply o-*soto-gari* instead.

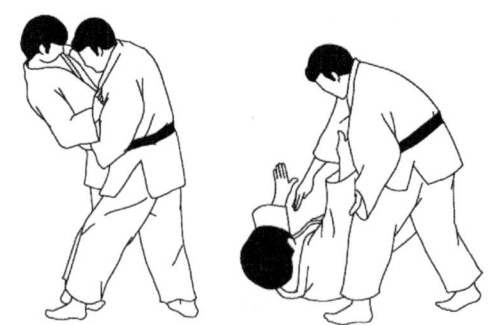

Chapter 4

Throws

- Leg and Foot Techniques
- Hand Techniques
- Shoulder Techniques
- Hip Techniques
- Sweeping Loin-Leg Techniques
- Rear Techniques
- Sacrifice Techniques

In this chapter are a series of guides to the most commonly taught throws.

Under present contest rules, the grabbing of legs is prohibited in competition, but may still be used in *randori* and *kata*.

Chapter 5 will introduce you to more complex throws and principles to follow on from Chapter 4.

Leg and Foot Throws

Core Technique – Leg Reap

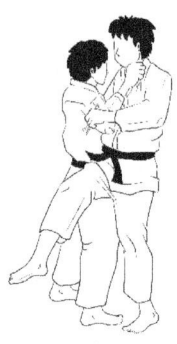

How to Apply Core Technique – Major Reap

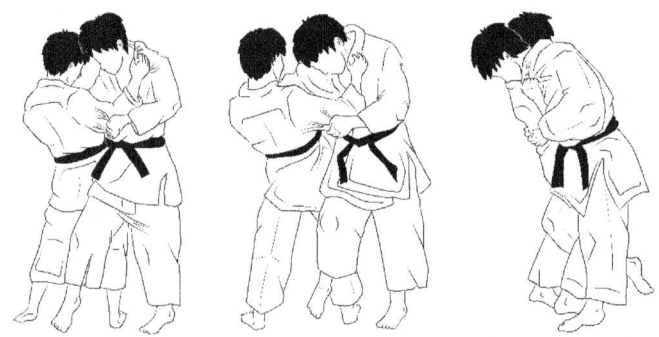

Pin opponent's weight onto their supporting leg then reap it.

Variations

O-soto-gari	O-uchi-gari
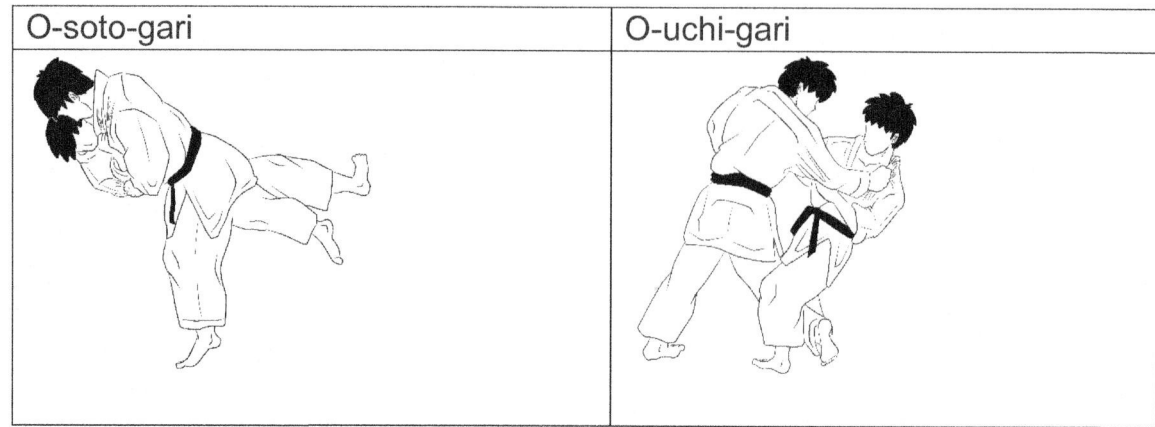	

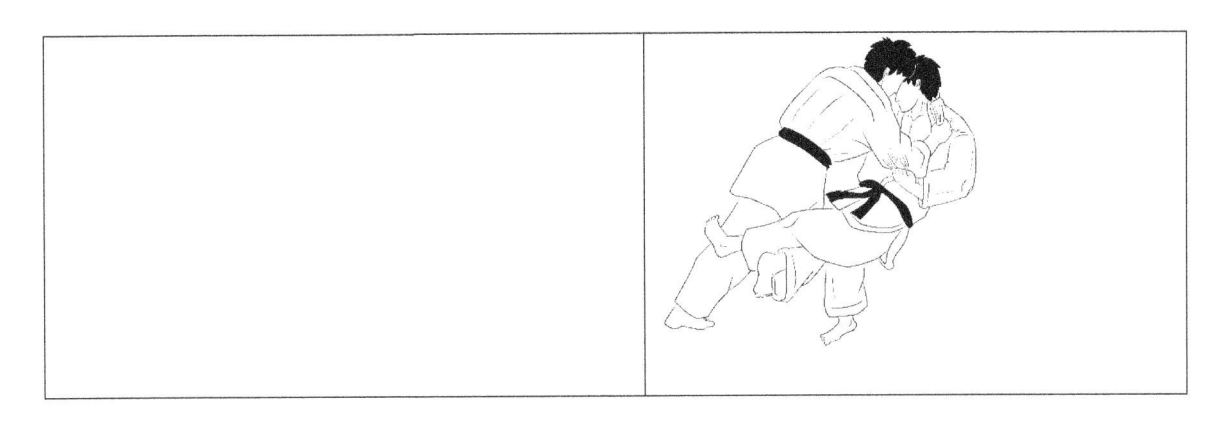

How to Apply Core Technique – Minor Reap

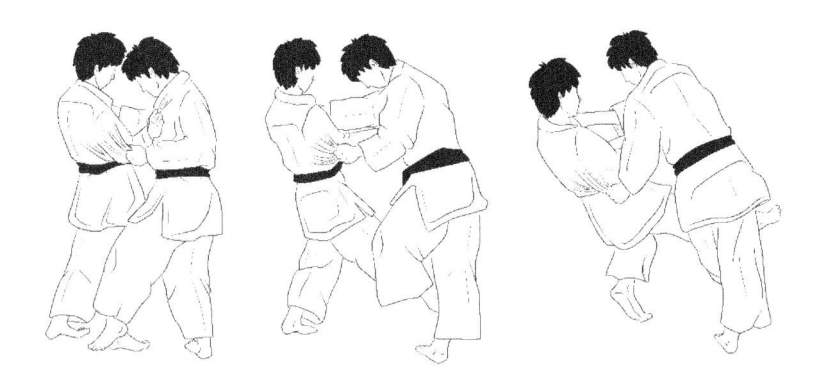

Variations – Pin and Rotate

Pin opponent on their supporting leg and rotate them over it. Sweep the non-weight bearing leg.

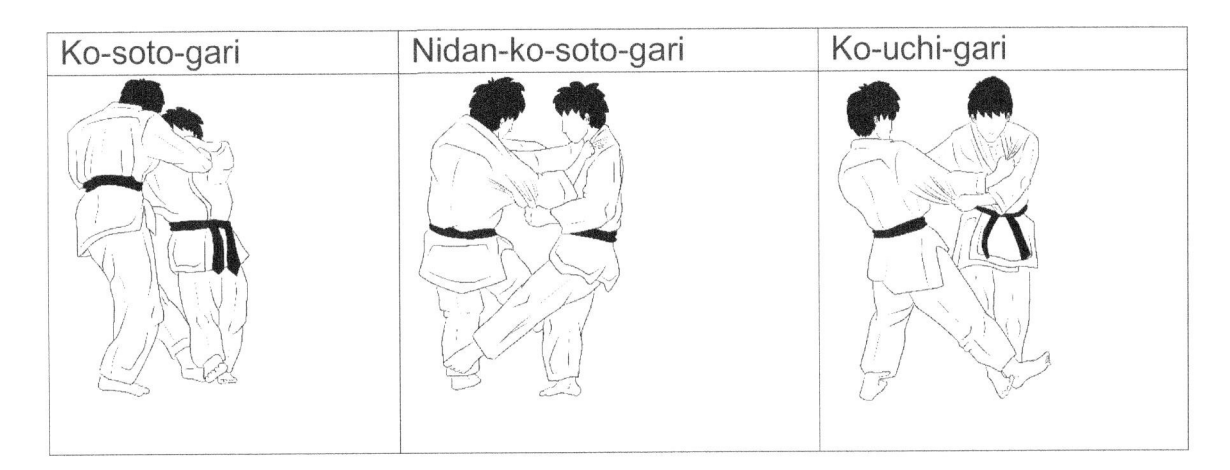

Ko-soto-gari	Nidan-ko-soto-gari	Ko-uchi-gari

Nidan-ko-soto-gari initially looks as though you are attacking the supporting leg. Rotating your opponent makes them switch weight so their weight bearing leg suddenly becomes non-weight bearing. Particularly if you first use *ko-soto-gari* then switch techniques to *nidan-ko-soto-gari*.

Variations – Foot Sweep

Sweep opponent's foot just after they move it and are about to place it on the ground to make it their weight bearing supporting leg.

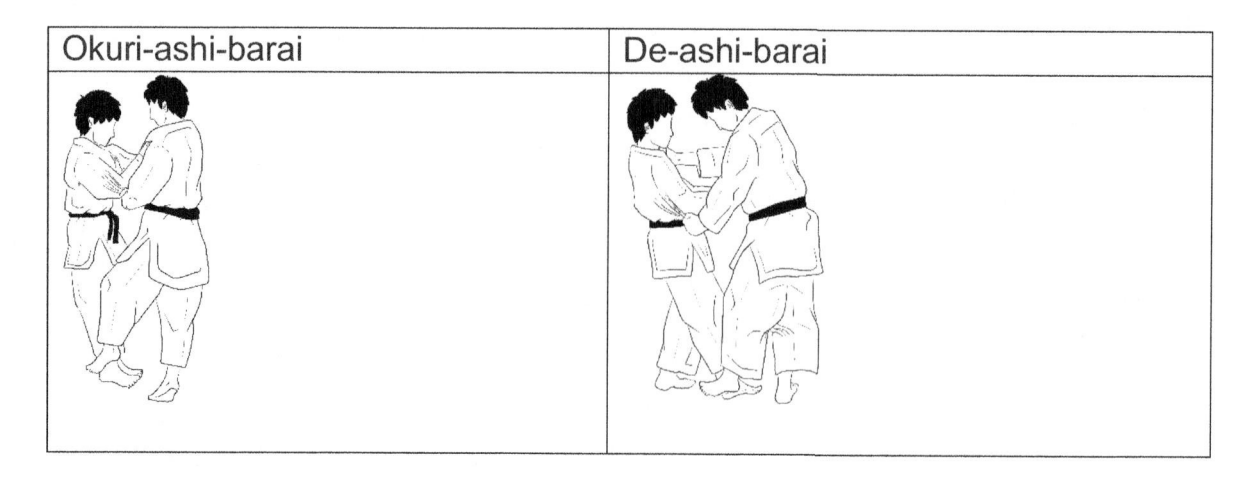

Okuri-ashi-barai	De-ashi-barai

Core Technique – Heel Trip

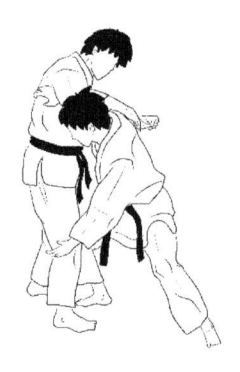

How to Apply Core Technique

Drive into opponent's body (almost like a rugby tackle) whilst reaping opponent's leg and wheeling over their upper body.

Principles of scoop and leg throws: Use scoop throw by gripping backs of opponent's thighs etc. when opponent upright, use leg throw when opponent in crouching position.

Variations

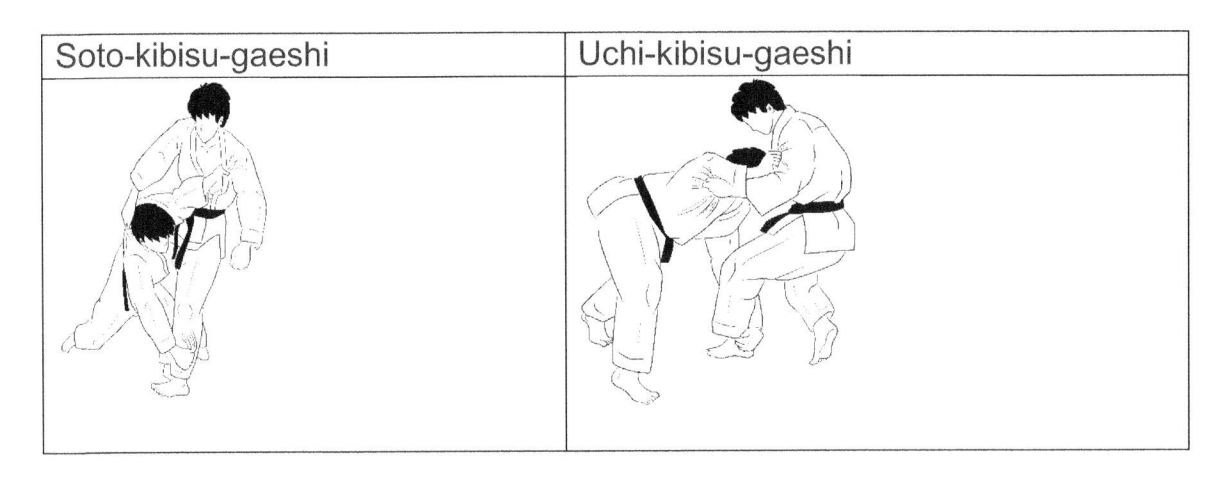

Soto-kibisu-gaeshi	Uchi-kibisu-gaeshi

Core Technique – Propping Drawing/Wheeling

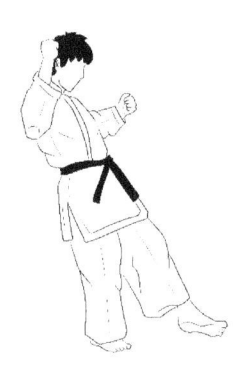

How to Apply Core Technique

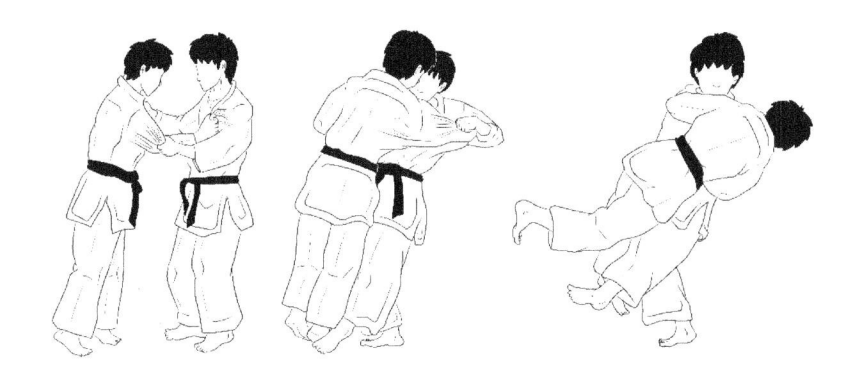

Move to the side and wheel your opponent so they trip over your outstretched foot (prop and roll).

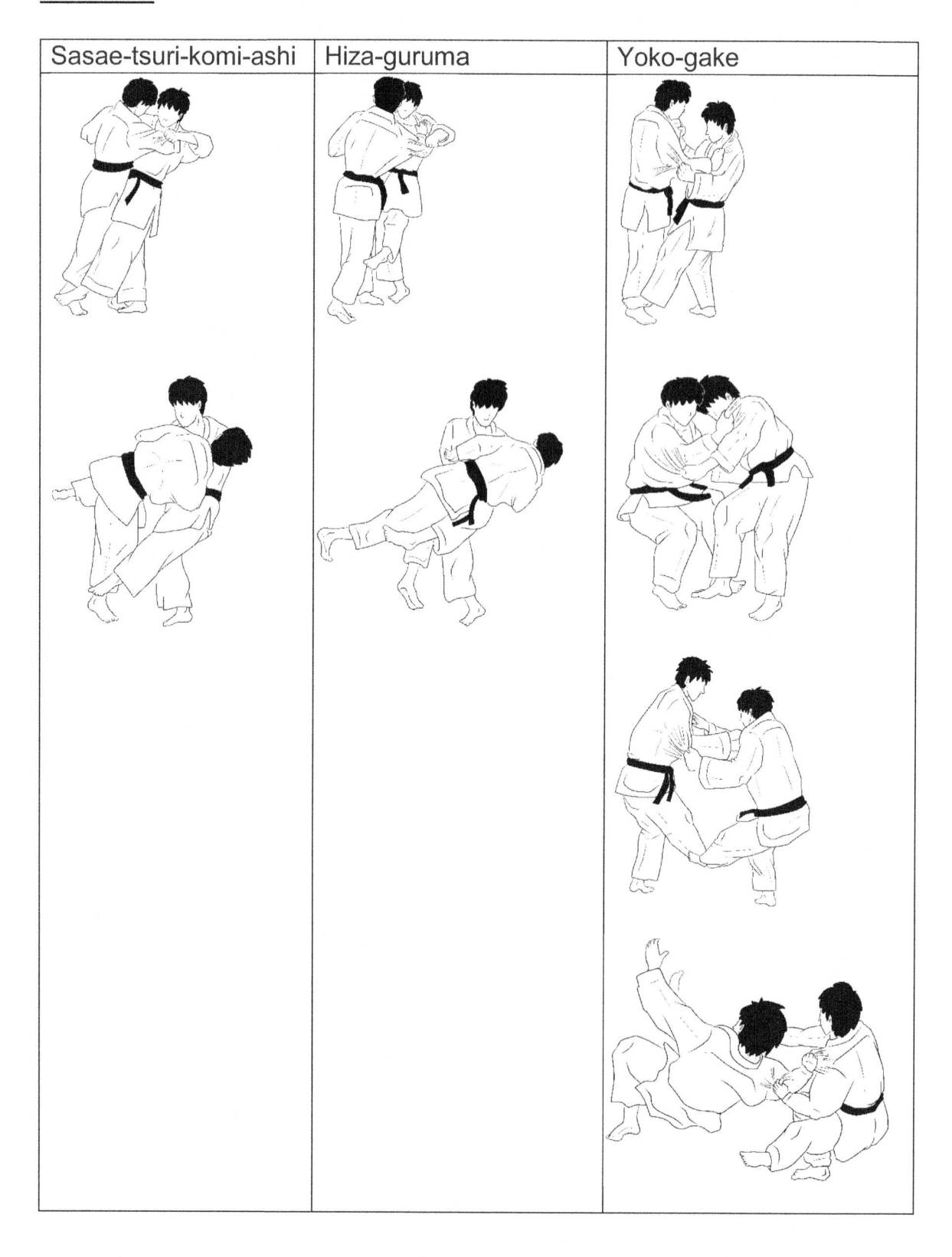

Variations

Sasae-tsuri-komi-ashi	Hiza-guruma	Yoko-gake

Hand Techniques

Core Technique – Shoulder Wheel

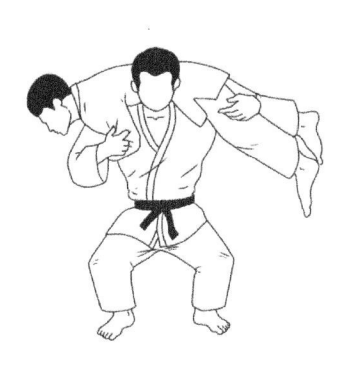

How to Apply Core Technique

Drop into a crouch position side on and at right angles to opponent. Drive your arm between opponent's legs and grip or lock-on round and behind opponent's thigh. At the same time, wrap opponent's arm across your shoulders and pull.

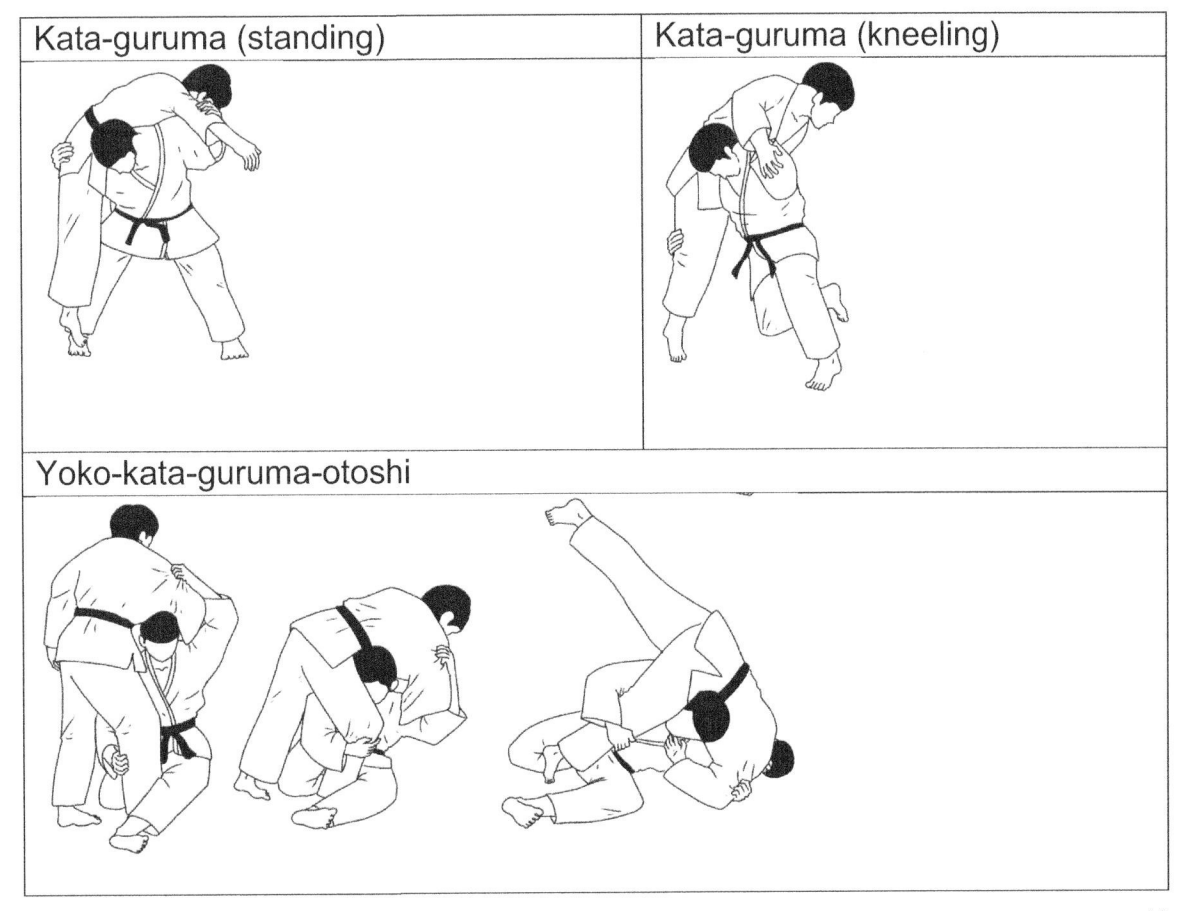

Variations

Kata-guruma (standing)	Kata-guruma (kneeling)

Yoko-kata-guruma-otoshi

Core Technique – Body Drop

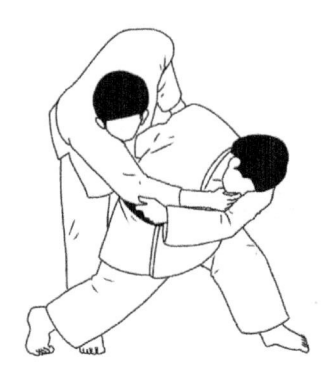

How to Apply Core Technique

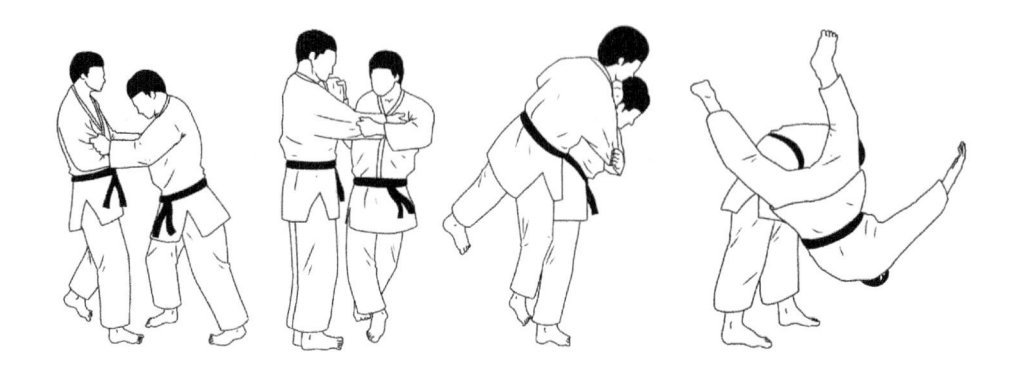

Seize opponent, lunge, then rotate opponent across your loin. Keep weight on your supporting leg, which is furthest from your opponent, this allows the other to   extend   as   your   body   drops.

Variations

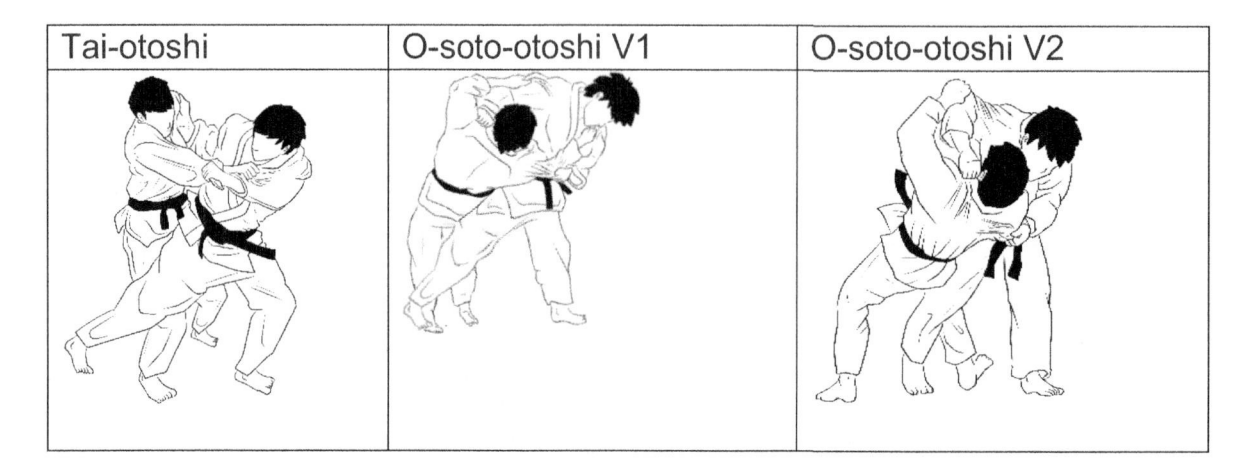

Tai-otoshi	O-soto-otoshi V1	O-soto-otoshi V2

If you apply *tai-otoshi* behind your opponent, you are applying *reverse body drop,* which is a variation on *o-soto-otoshi*.

Core Technique – Floating Drop

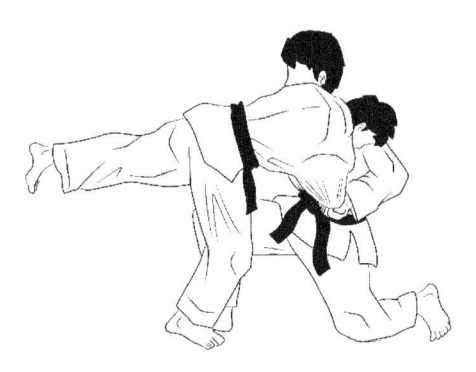

How to Apply Core Technique

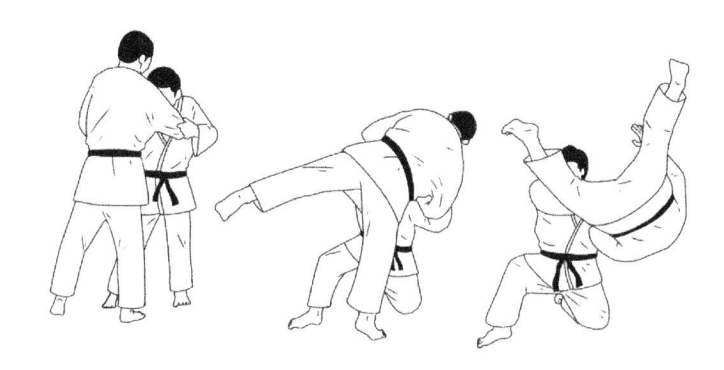

Drop backwards to gain momentum and wheel over opponent using sleeve and lapel grips.

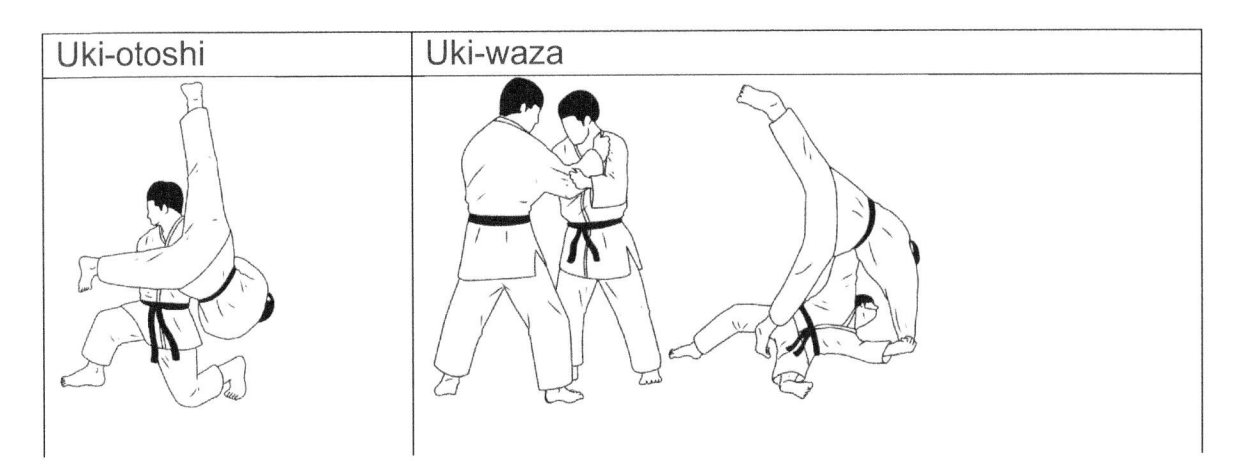

Variations

Uki-otoshi	Uki-waza

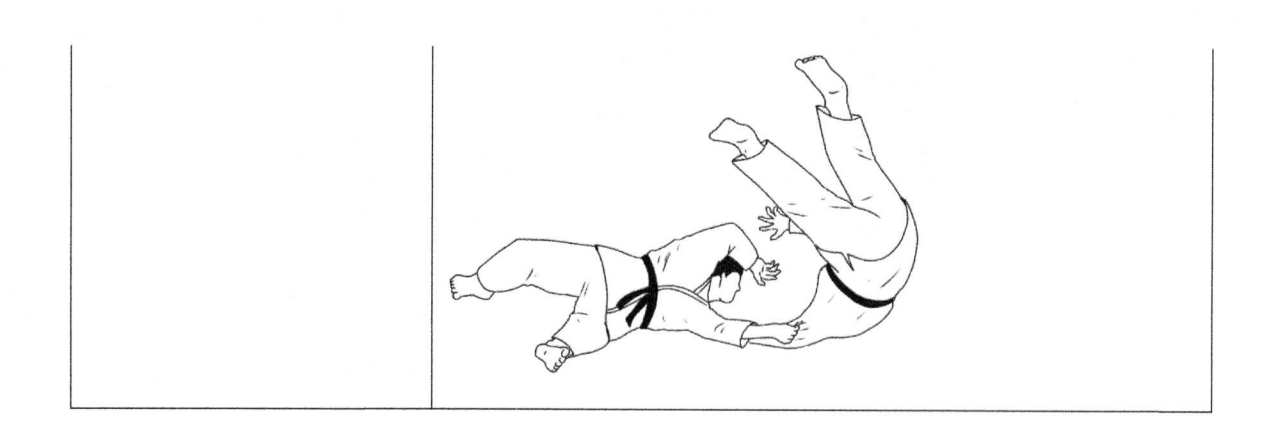

Shoulder Throws

Core Technique

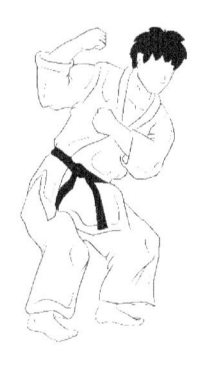

How to Apply Core Technique

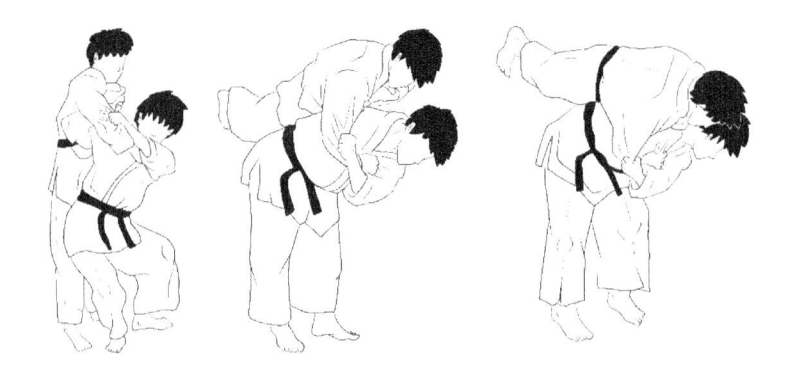

Stand between opponent's feet and roll your opponent over your shoulder with a winding motion to draw them around.

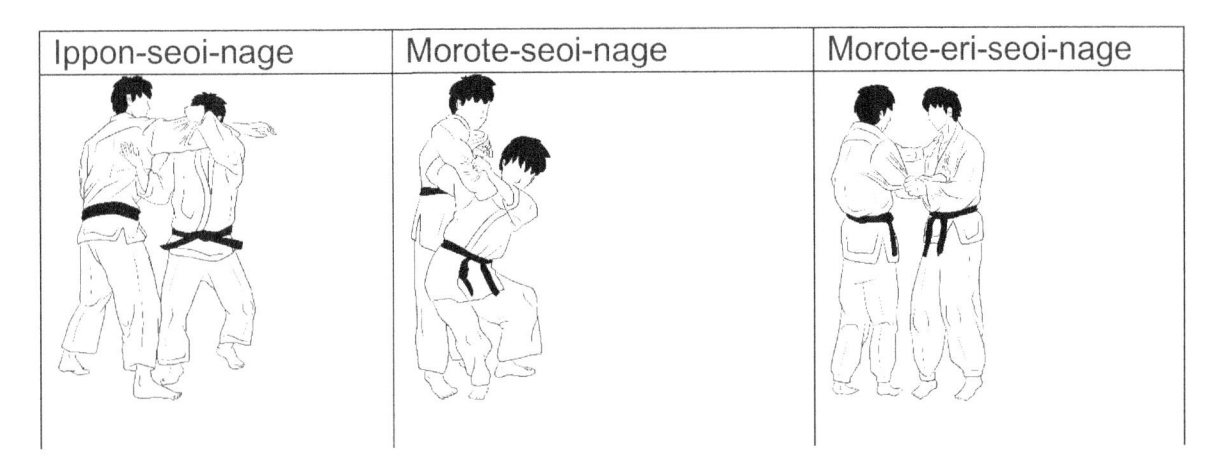

Variations

Ippon-seoi-nage	Morote-seoi-nage	Morote-eri-seoi-nage

| Seoi-otoshi | Ryo-hiza-seoi-otoshi | |

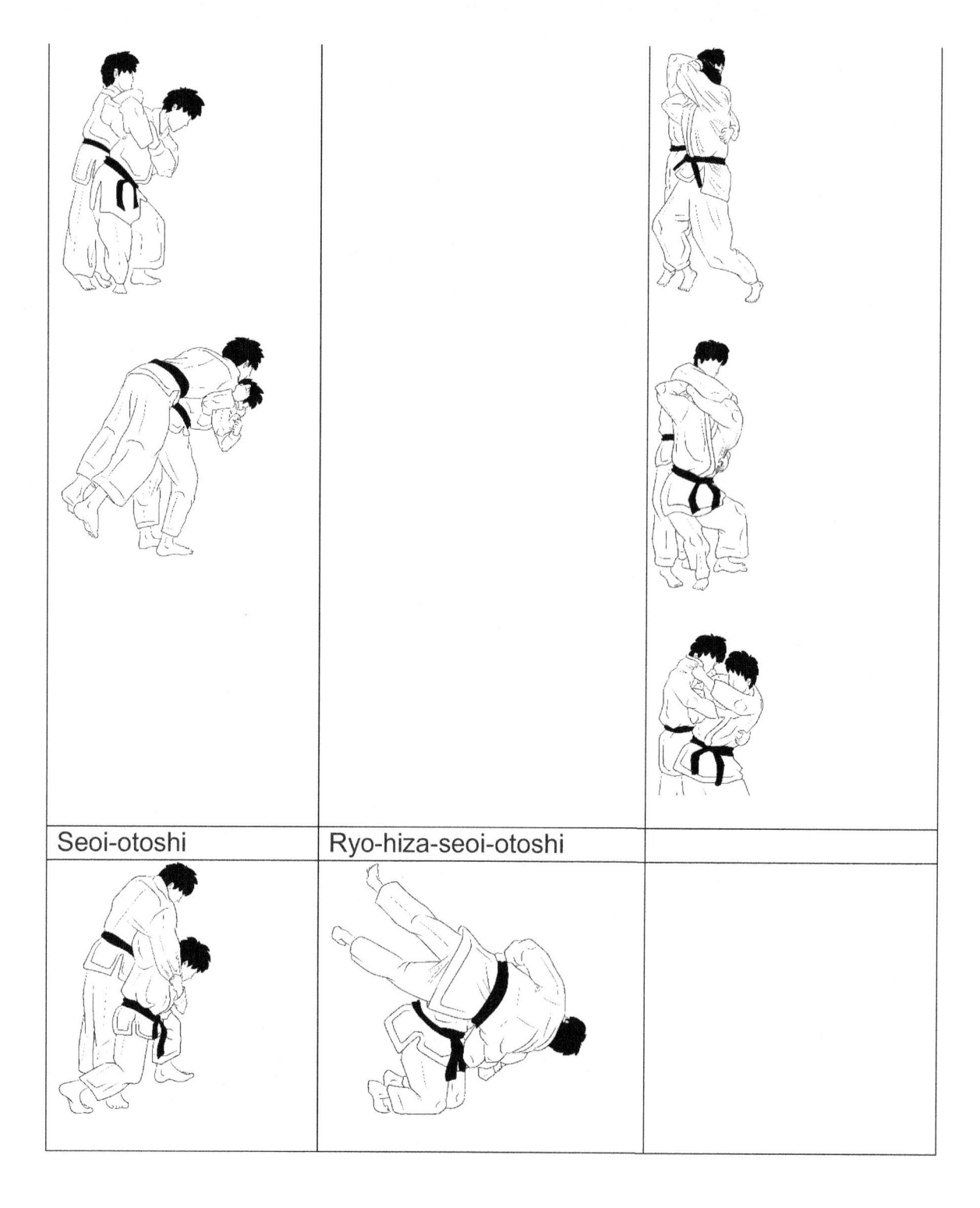

Hip Techniques

Core Technique

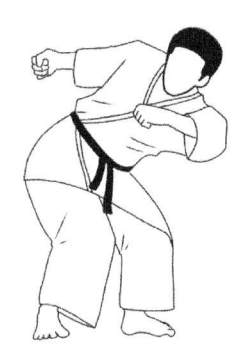

How to Apply Core Technique

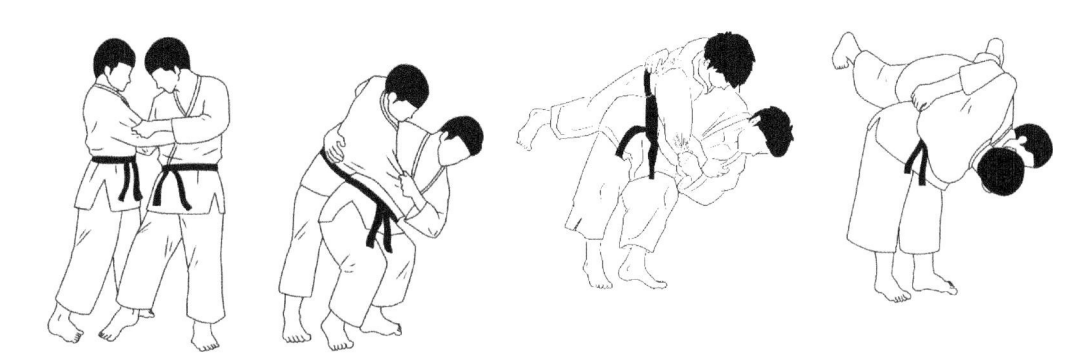

Stand between opponent's feet and roll your opponent over your hip.

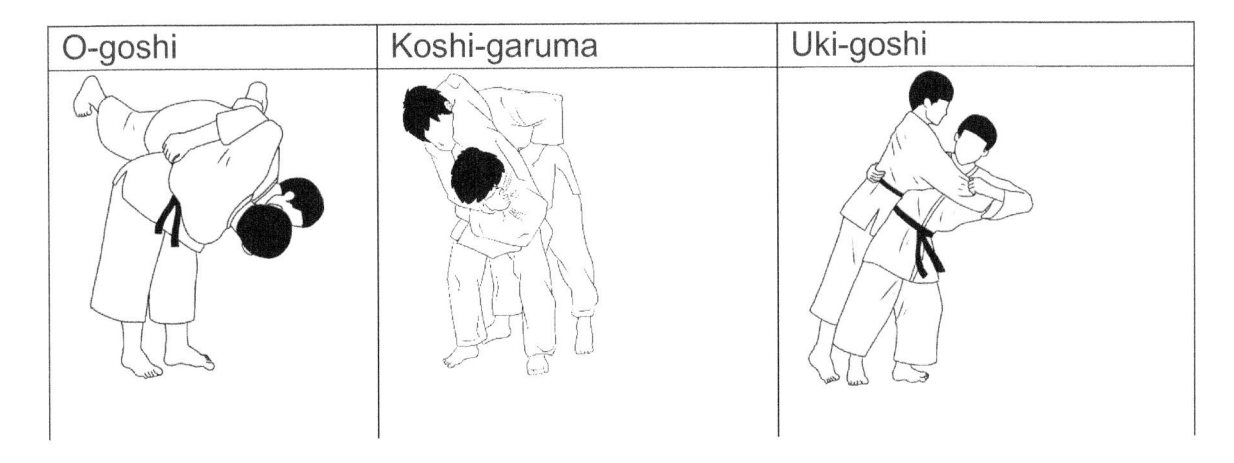

Variations

O-goshi	Koshi-garuma	Uki-goshi

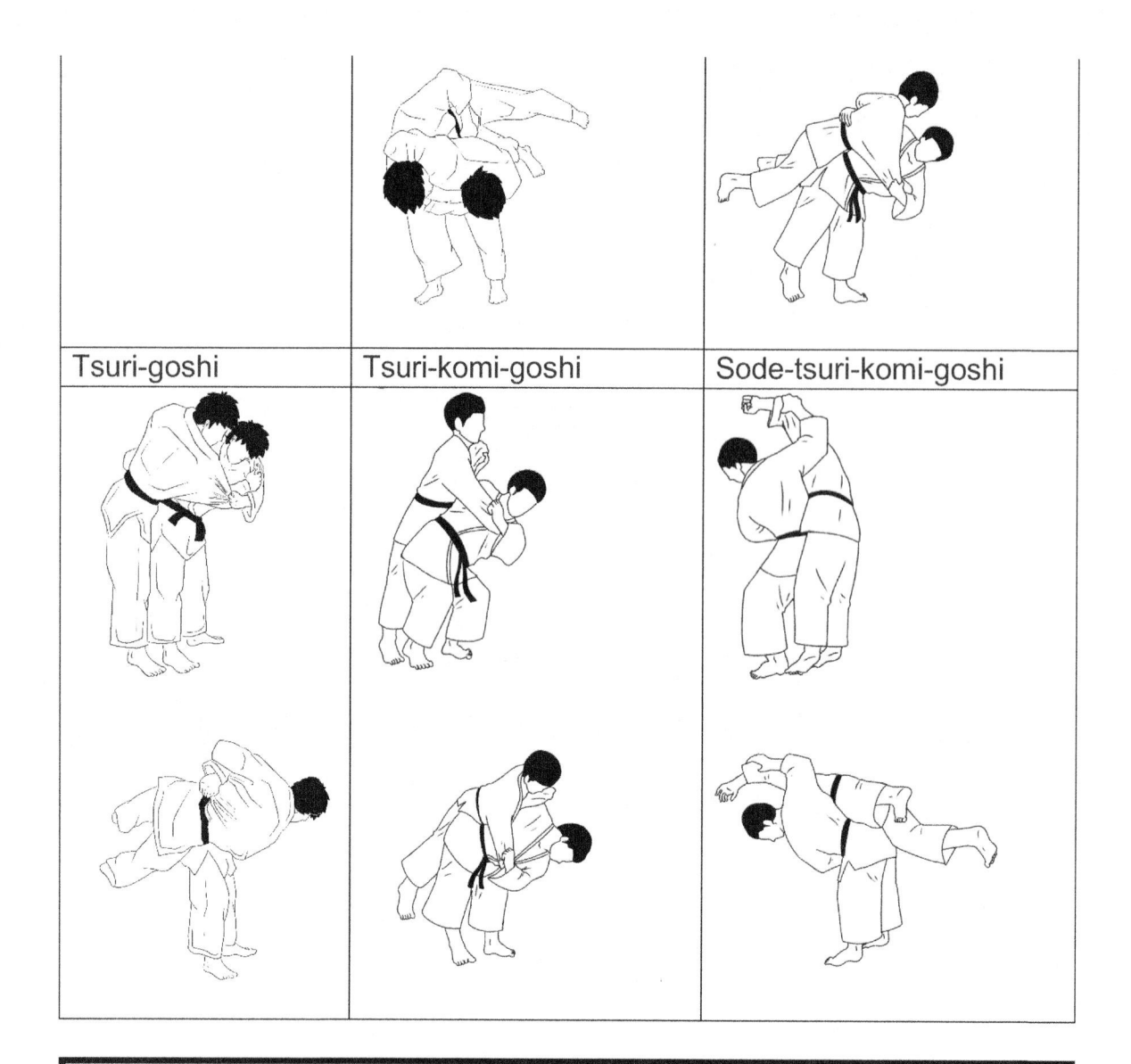

Tsuri-goshi	Tsuri-komi-goshi	Sode-tsuri-komi-goshi

> *O-goshi* is a key movement principle to learn; I would say a key foundation technique. Once you have mastered it, the body movement is used in many *judo* throws. For example, change the arm grip and you have *ippon-seoi-nage*. This idea of modular parts of throws is set out in Chapter 5.

If you stand beside your opponent (instead of between their feet), whilst facing over your opponent's shoulder (instead of facing the same way as them) and apply *uki-goshi;* you are doing the *reverse hip throw* on them. This is sometimes known as a variation on *ushiro-goshi*.

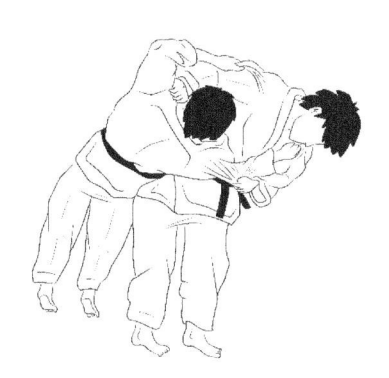

Sweeping Loin/Leg Techniques

Core Technique

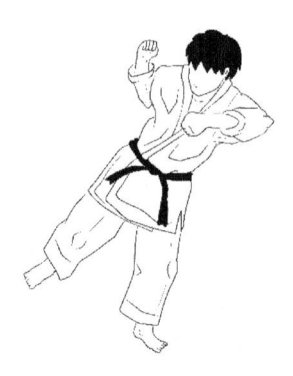

How to Apply Core Technique

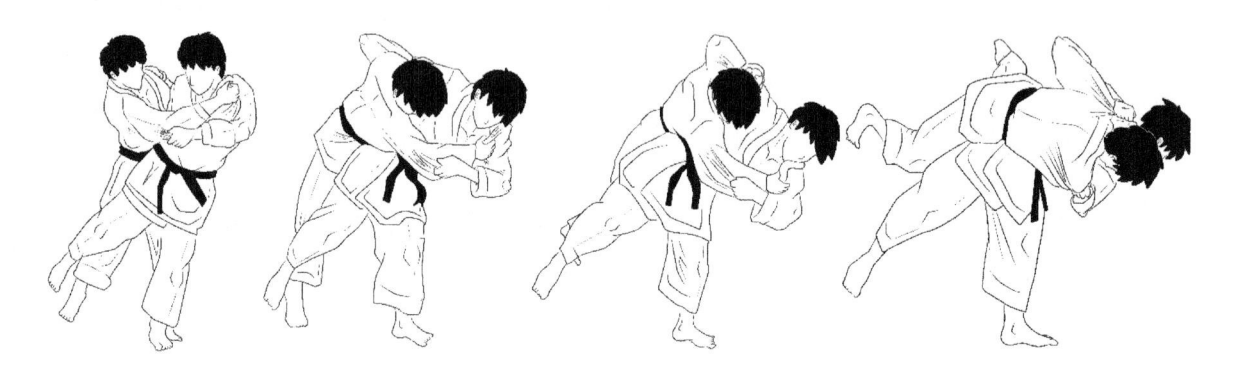

Stand between opponent's feet and roll your opponent over your loin. Sweep back your leg more like a back kick than a reap (as used in *o-soto-gari*).

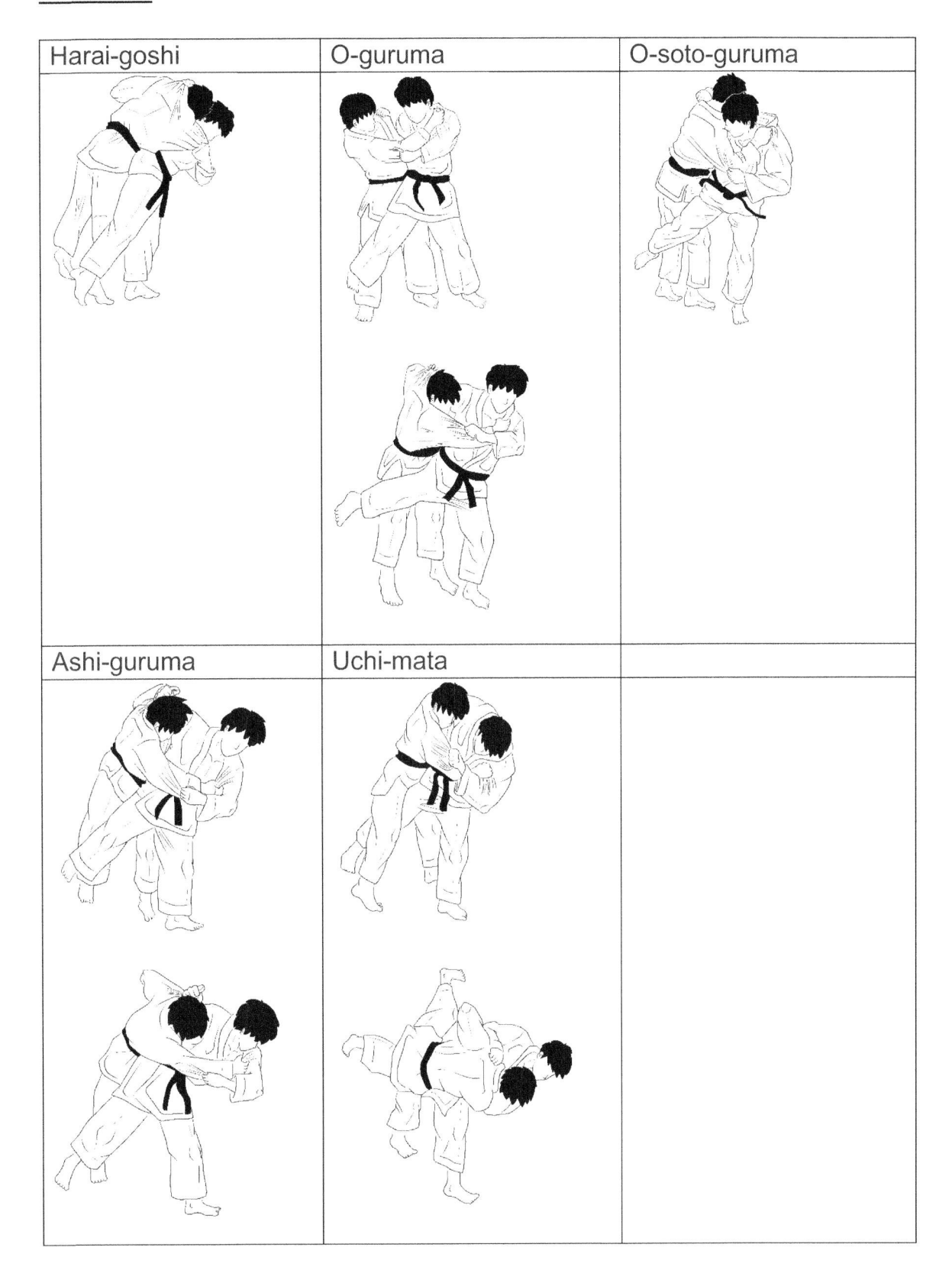

Variations

Harai-goshi	O-guruma	O-soto-guruma

Ashi-guruma	Uchi-mata	

Rear Techniques

Core Technique

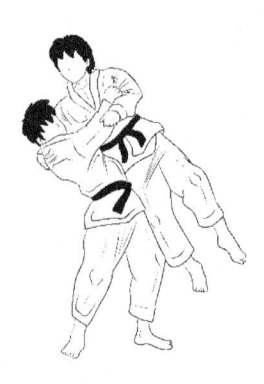

How to Apply Core Technique

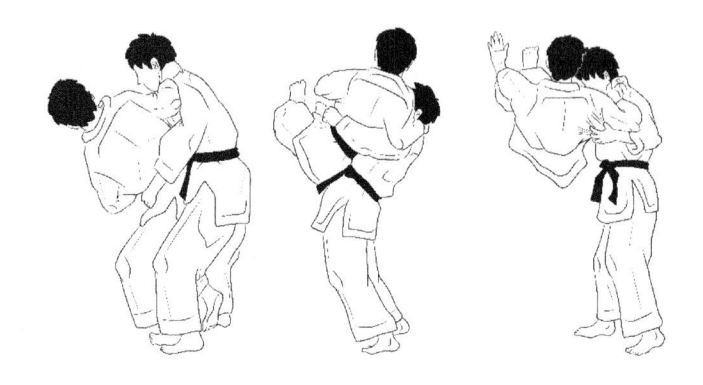

Stand behind opponent and roll them over your hip whilst thrusting diagonally upwards in the direction your opponent is turning. (This technique wells work as a counter throw such as when your opponent is trying to use *o-goshi*.)

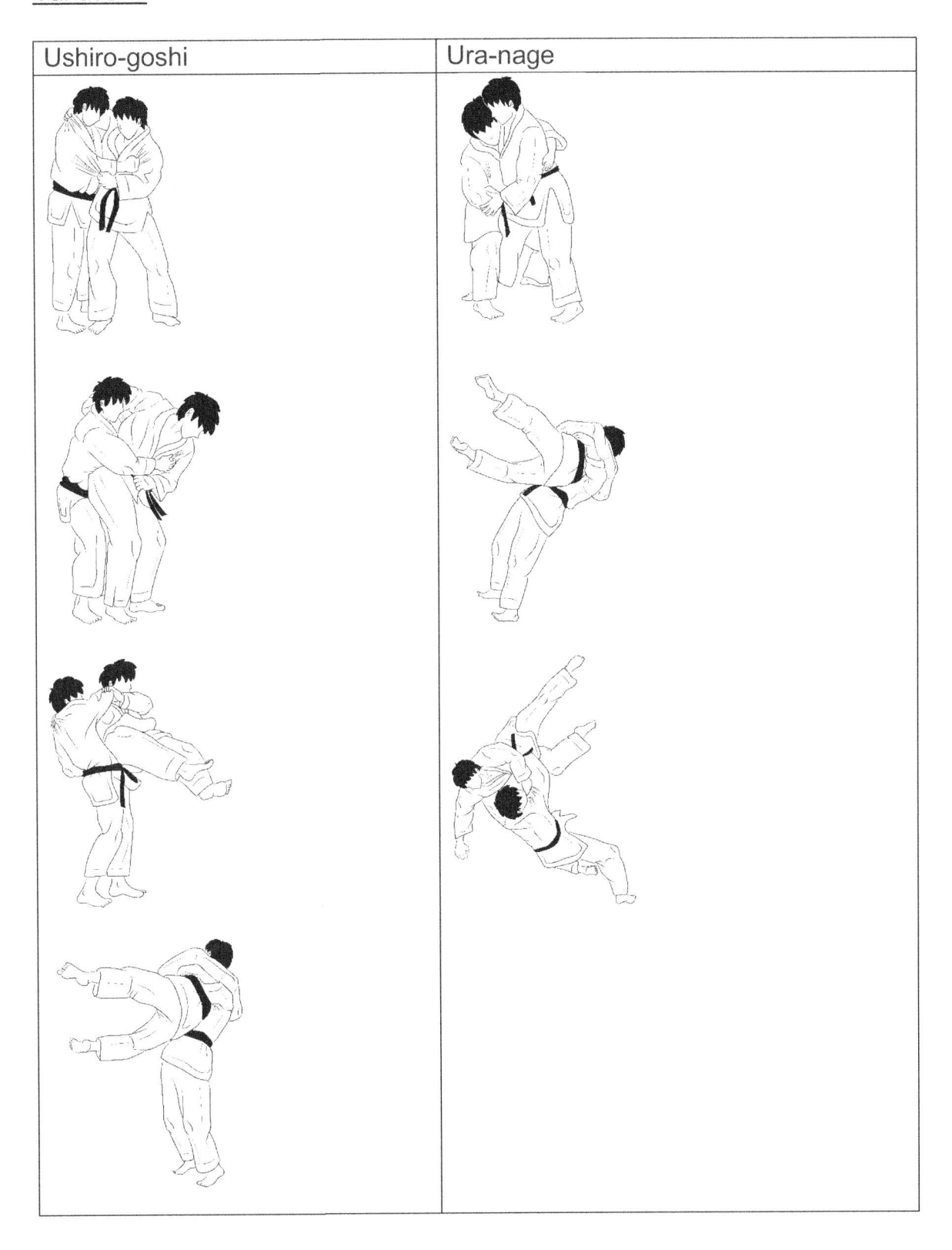

Variations

Ushiro-goshi	Ura-nage

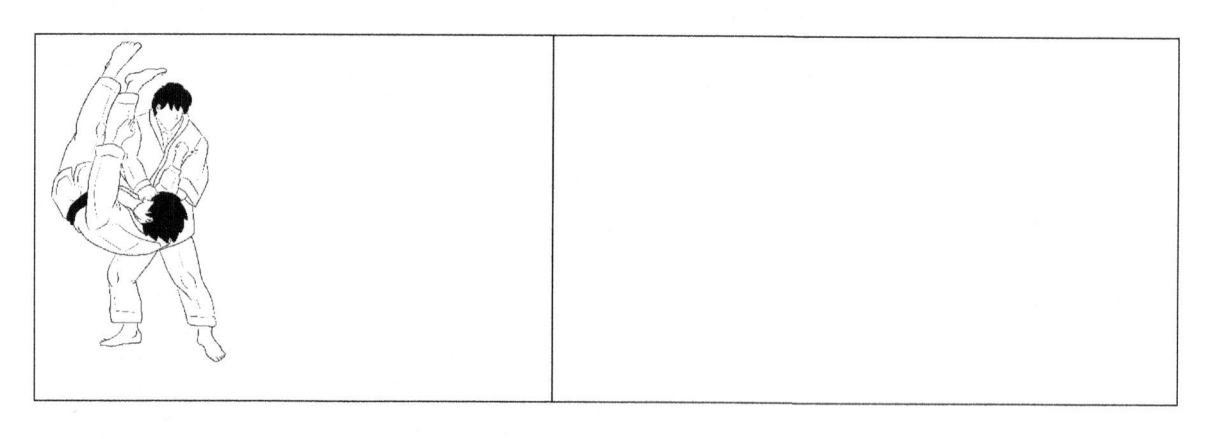

Ura-nage picture 1 shows another possible position for applying the throw.

Sacrifice Techniques

When doing sacrifice throws you will have to get right under the other person to throw them over you. Almost as though the person doing the throw and the person being thrown swap places.

> Get right under the other person to throw them over you.

Core Technique – Circle Throw

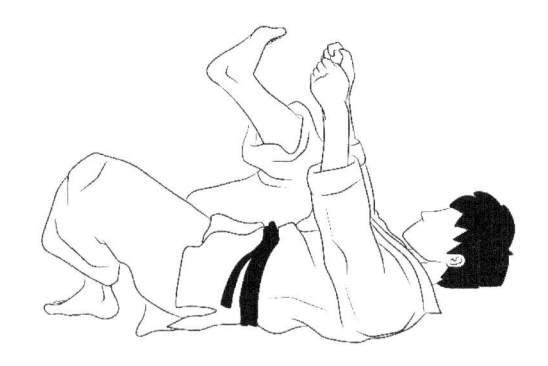

<u>How to Apply Core Technique</u>

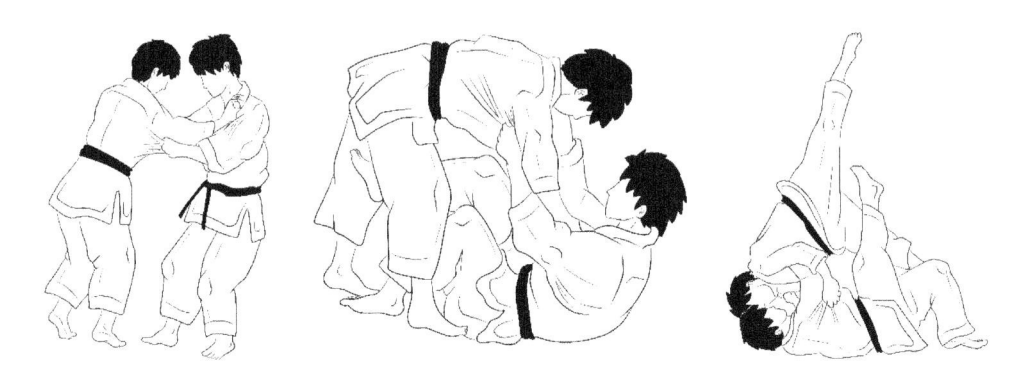

Drop between opponent's feet and roll opponent over yourself, using your foot as a fulcrum.

Variations

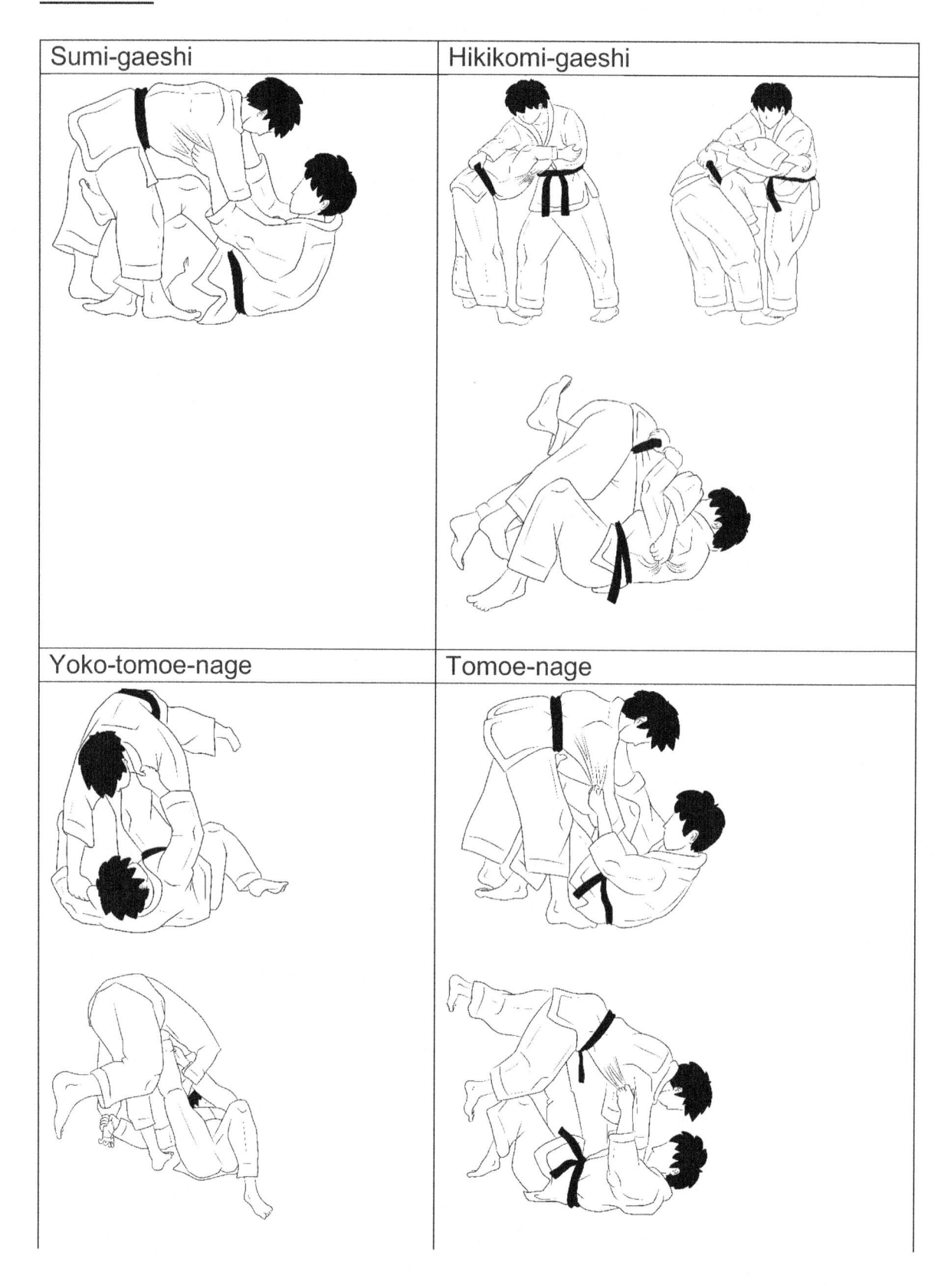

Sumi-gaeshi	Hikikomi-gaeshi

Yoko-tomoe-nage	Tomoe-nage

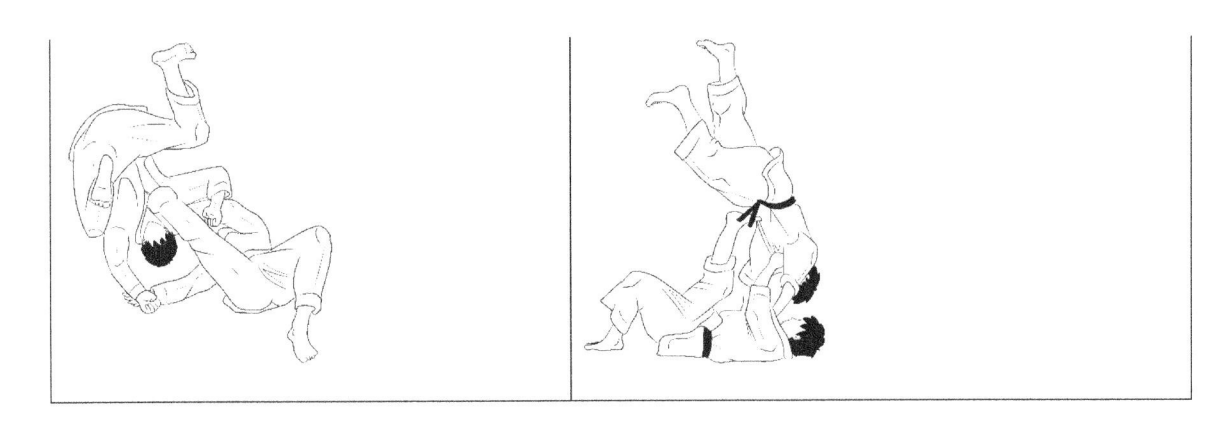

Core Technique – Drop Throws

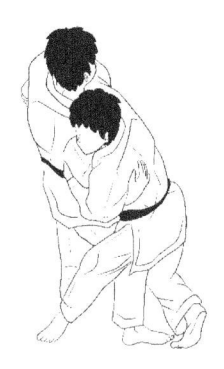

How to Apply Core Technique

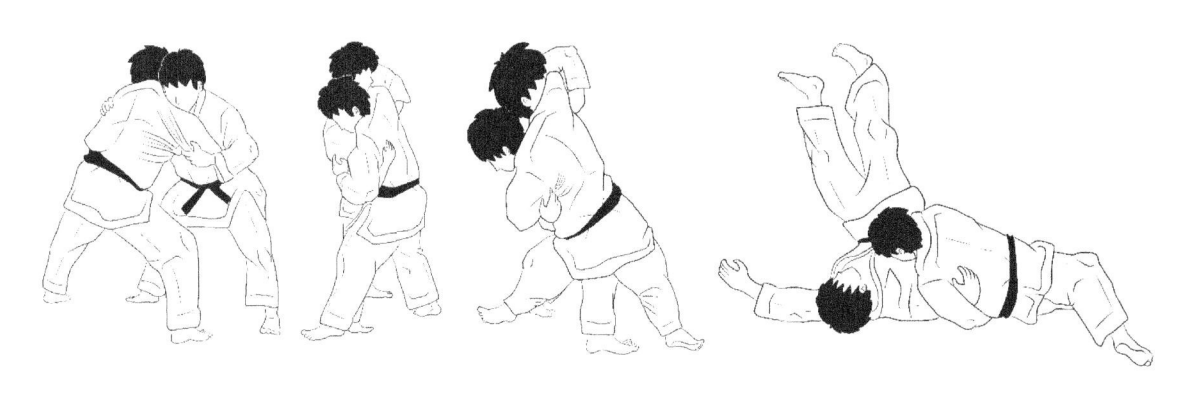

Drop onto your side at opponent's feet and roll opponent over yourself.

| Tani-otoshi | Yoko otoshi |

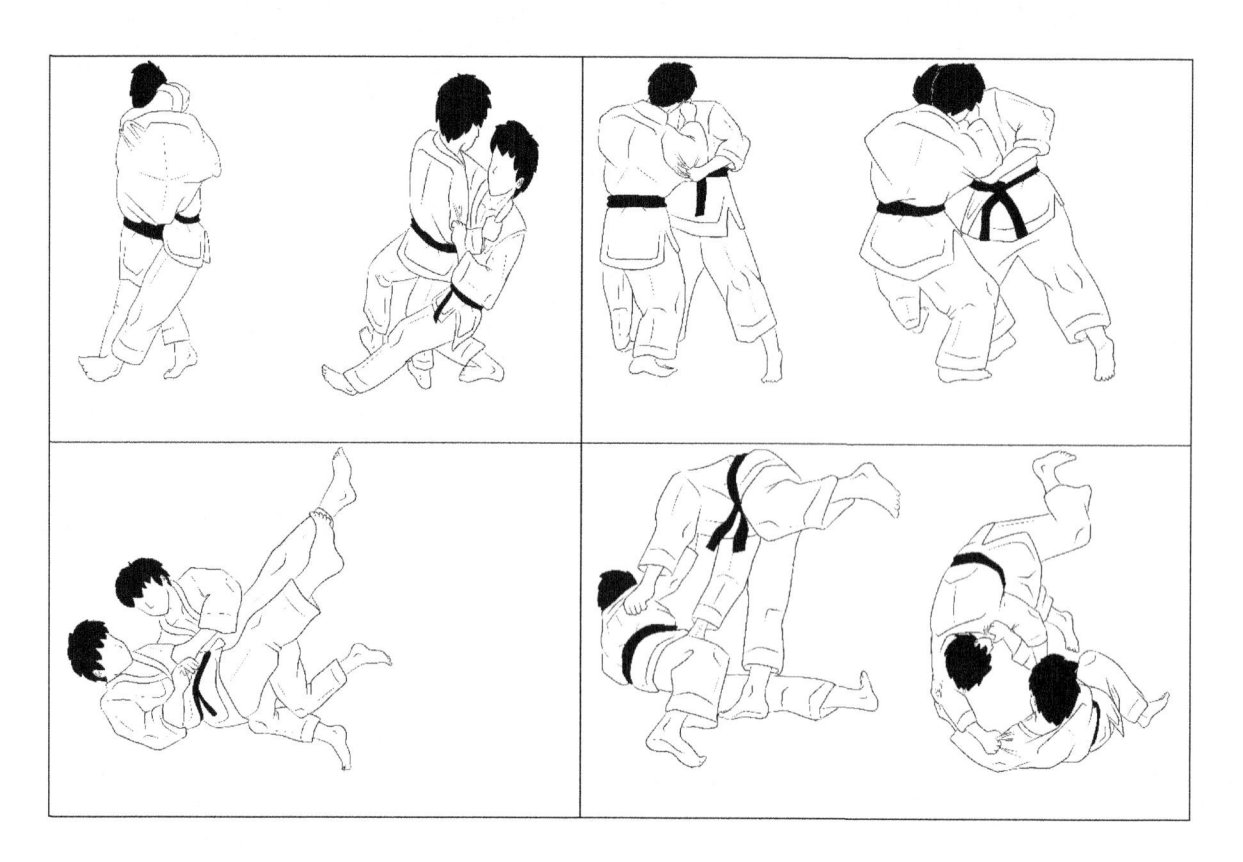

Core Technique – Side Rolling Throws

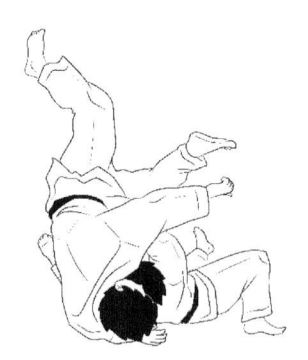

How to Apply Core Technique

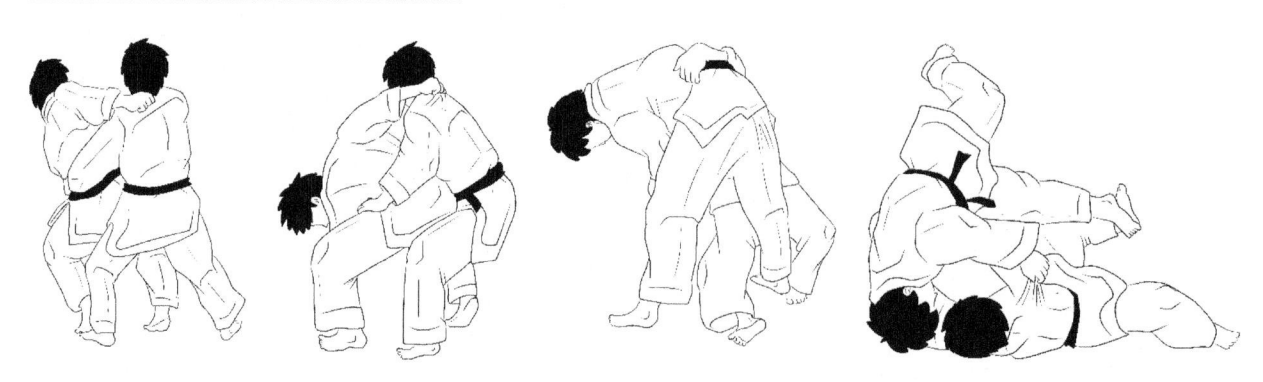

Drop onto your side at opponent's feet and roll opponent over yourself.

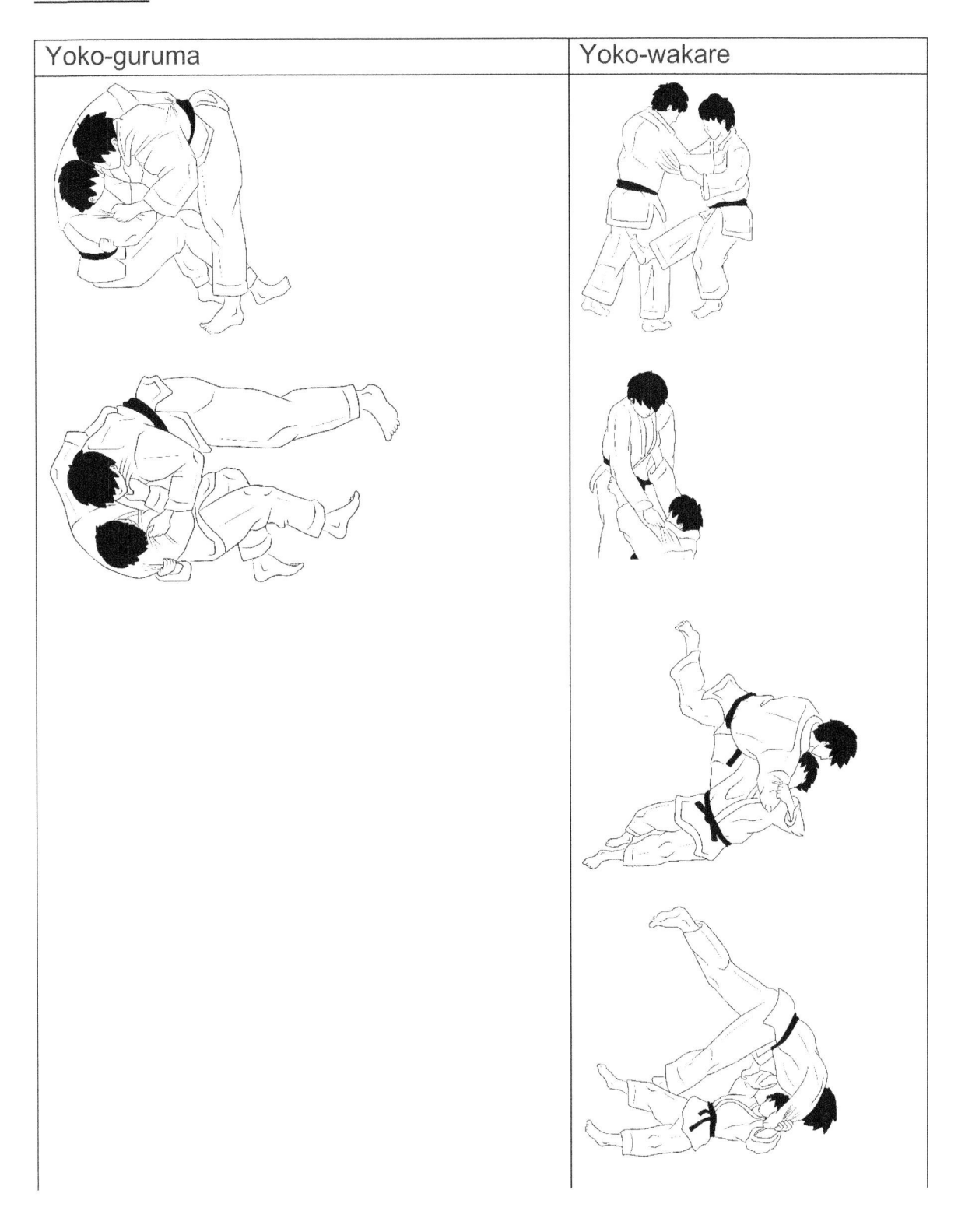

Variations

Yoko-guruma	Yoko-wakare

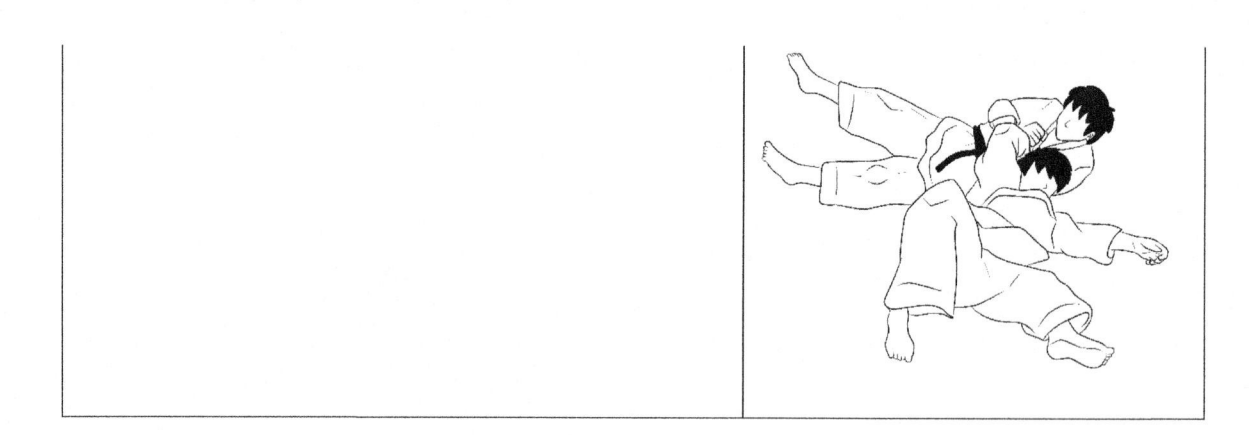

Chapter 5

Modular Parts of Throws

- Kata
- Modular Parts of Throws

Kata

There are two principle ways of practising *judo*: *Kata* and *randori*. *Kata* is a formal system of pre-arranged/stylised movements. Randori meaning "free practice" is almost 'learn through play' (i.e. practise what you have just been taught or know already).

The application of *judo* movements can be learnt in a style people normally associate with *aikido*, rather than the grip fighting style sometimes seen on television/YouTube/Olympics. For example, *ju-no-kata* could be described as a *kata* of suppleness for exercise and learning *judo* principles through movement.

Originally there were ten *katas* that could be learnt:
1. *Nage-no-kata* (forms of throwing). Five groups of three throws illustrate different aspects of *nage-waza* (the ideal application/demonstration of how to apply throws): *Te-waza, koshi-waza, ashi-waza, ma-sutemi-waza* and *yoko-sutemi-waza*.
2. *Katame-no-kata* (forms of groundwork). Fifteen techniques can be learnt/applied, five from each of the three sub-divisions of *katame-waza*: *Osaekomi-waza, shime-waza* and *kansetsu-waza*. Similar in intent to *nage-no-kata*, but focused on the fundamental techniques of control whatever the initial and final positions.
3. *Ju-no-kata* (forms of gentleness and flexibility). A sequence of fifteen reactions to attack (i.e. practice methods of attack and defence) arranged in three sets to illustrate the principle of *ju* (gentleness, suppleness, yielding skill e.g. pull when your opponent pushes). Some focus is put on displacement of your opponent's energy, but not as much as in *itsutsu-no-kata*.
4. *Go-no-seno kata* (forms of counter-throwing). A sequence of twelve attacks in which the demonstrator snatches the initiative from an attacker (i.e. uses counter attacks in response to initial attacks).
5. *Kime-no-kata* (forms of decision/decisive techniques). Twenty disabling moves arranged in two sets (eight and twelve respectively) variously directed against an unarmed attacker or one armed with knife or sword. Originally, this was called the *"Kata of Self-Defence"*.
6. *Koshiki-no-kata* (ancient forms of throwing). Stylised demonstration of twenty-one methods of attack and defence derived from *ju jitsu* methods, which preceded *judo*.

7. *Itsutsu-no-kata* (form of five concepts). A kata which attempts to capture and portray the precise moment at which presence of mind causes the downfall of an opponent (i.e. when you can seize the initiative and control your opponent). These forms express the mechanism of attack and defence in a way that tries to synthesise the fundamental forms of *tai-sabaki* (body movement) and control direction of your opponent's energy. It consists of just five sequences of movement. This *kata* is more esoteric than *ju-no-kata*.
8. *Seiryoku-zenyo-kokumin-taiiku* (national physical exercise based on the principle of maximum efficiency). The complete repertoire involves thirty-six set pieces in three groups: Sixteen striking and kicking actions, ten attacks and ten pliable responses.
9. *Goshin-jutsu-no-kata* (self-defence *kata* for men).
10. *Joshi-goshin-ho-kata* (self-defence *kata* for women). This is a kata of eighteen movements in three parts: Eight basic patterns, five methods of escape and five methods of retaliation. It is a *kata* that is rarely taught today.

Opinion is split between different *judo* bodies on how many *kata* should be taught. For example:
- *Joshi-goshin-ho-kata* appears to have been replaced by *goshin-jutsu kata* as *judo's* self-defence *kata* for all *judoka* (i.e. no longer two *kata* split into self-defence *kata* for men or women).
    - This consists of an "unarmed section" and a "weapons section". The "unarmed section" consists of twelve techniques while the "weapons section" consists of nine techniques.
- *Gonosen-no-kata* is not an officially recognized *judo kata*, but its importance is recognised by its inclusion in Kawaishi's "*The Complete Seven Katas of Judo*". It is mainly practiced by western nations, and often each country has its unique portfolio of techniques. The *British Judo Association* recently modified its version on the BJA website.
- Details in table below showing the number of *katas* to be taught varies between seven and nine.

International Judo Federation	British Judo Association	British Judo Council	Kodokan Judo Institute
1. Goshin-jutsu-kata 2. Itsutsu-no-kata	1. Gonosen-no-kata 2. Itsutsu-no-kata 3. Ju-no-kata	1. Katame-no-kata 2. Nage-no-kata	1. Nage-no-kata

3. Ju-no-kata 4. Katame-no-kata 5. Kime-no-kata 6. Koshiki-no-kata 7. Nage-no-kata	4. Katame-no-kata 5. Kime-no-kata 6. Kodokan goshin-jutsu kata 7. Koshiki-no-kata 8. Nage-no-kata	3. Ju-no-kata 4. Goshin-jutsu-kata 5. Kime-no-kata 6. Itsutsu-no-kata 7. Kaeshi-no-kata or Go-no-seno	2. Katame-no-kata 3. Kime-no-kata 4. Ju-no-kata 5. Kodokan goshin-jutsu kata 6. Itsutsu-no-kata 7. Koshiki-no-kata 8. Seiryoku-zenyo-kokumin-taiiku 9. Kodomo-no-kata

> *Kata* in *judo* teaches how to attack, how to defend and when to do so as a sequence of pre-arranged moves. The techniques should be applied with commitment, in the same style as 'three step sparring' as used in other martial arts.

Kata in *judo* teaches the principles that make techniques work. You can then apply these principles in many different ways through different throws by changing:
- Hand grips.
- Modular parts of throws.

Throws are made up from modular parts: Arms, bodies and legs. The different parts can be combined in different ways. For example, *hane-goshi* and *maki-komi* in combination make *hane-maki-komi*.

Hane-goshi	Soto-maki-komi	Hane-maki-komi
+		=

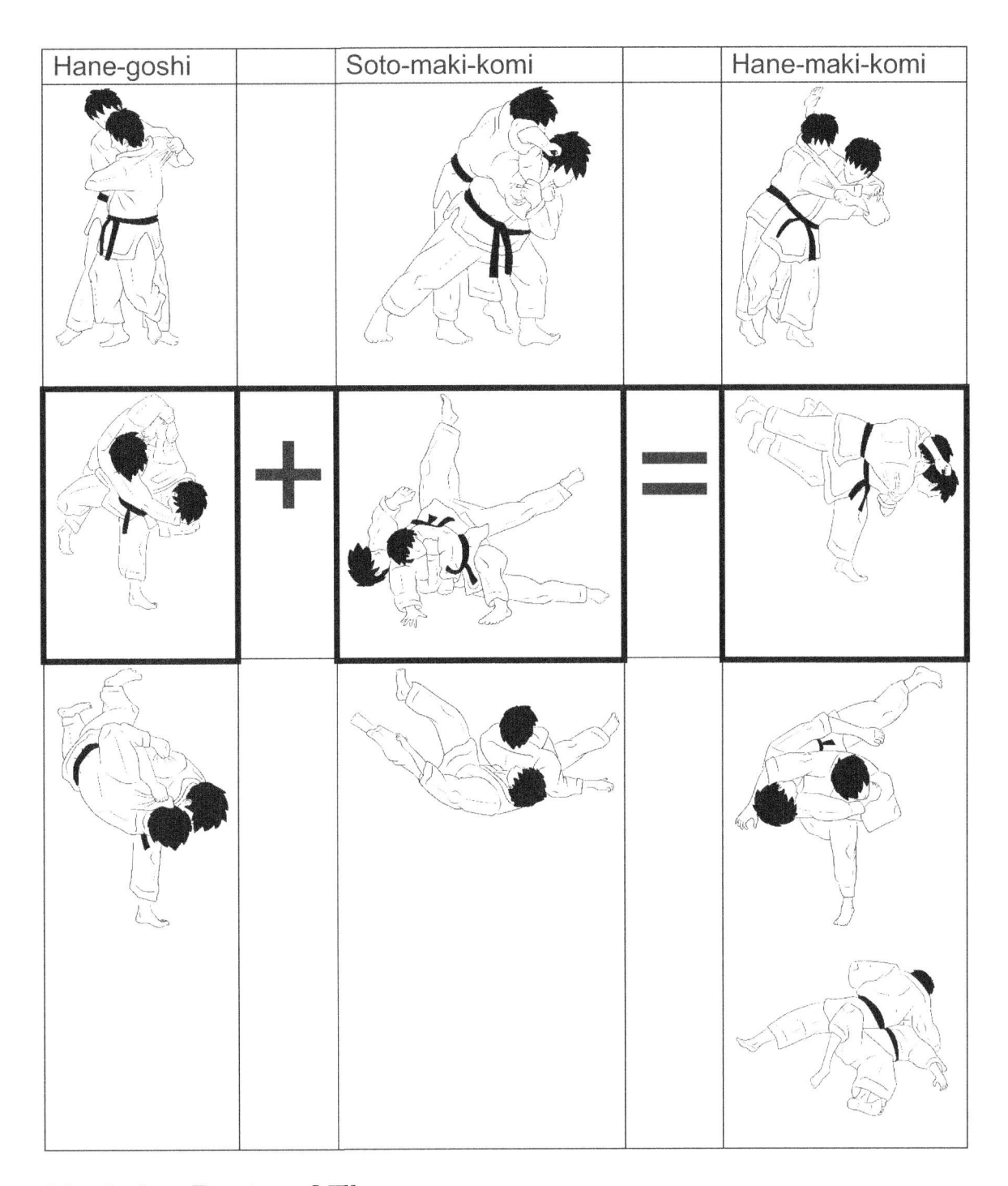

Modular Parts of Throws

You can now understand why I suggest that by using one principle in different positions, you can get several different throws from the same technique. Sometimes by using the same movement, other times by changing modular parts of the throw: Arms, bodies and legs (i.e. grips, movement and position).

You can use different limbs for the same actions. For example, reaping:

- Legs:
    - *O-soto-gari.*
    - *Kata-hiza-te-ouchi-gake-ashi-dori.*
- Arms:
    - *Kata-uchi-ashi-dori.*
    - *Morote-gari (as shown below).*

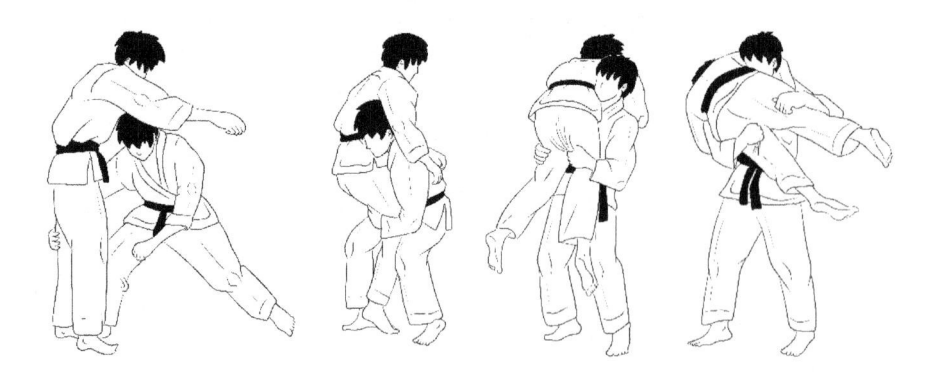

You may need to change the direction of the throw when applying the principle in different ways.

Examples of Modular Throw Components

Variation on a theme

O-soto-gari (reap) > *O-soto-gake* (scoop), or *Ko-soto-gari* (reap) > *Ko-soto-gake* (scoop). Instead of reaping your opponent's supporting leg at the base of the calf, make a scooping action with your heel to the back of opponent's knee. (You can use the back of your own knee instead of a heel if opponent is standing close.)

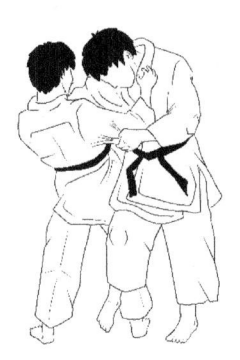

| Ko-soto-gake | O-soto-gake |

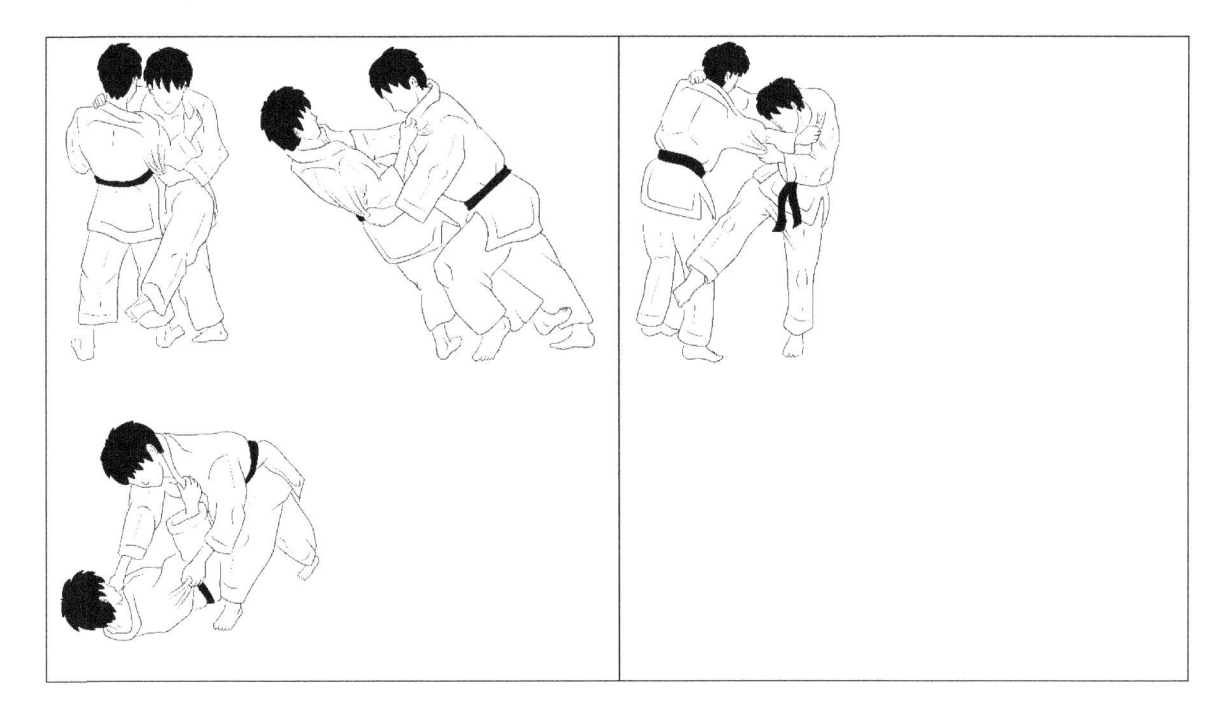

You can combine *sasae-tsuri-komi-ashi* with a *forward leg sweep* to make a combined sweeping drawing ankle throw: *Harai-tsuri-komi-ashi*. With *sasae-tsuri-komi-ashi*, the idea is to move to the side and wheel your opponent so they trip over your outstretched foot. With *harai-tsuri-komi-ashi*, the idea is to move forward, drive your outstretched foot forward to sweep your opponent's supporting leg as they step, then wheel your opponent so he/she trips over your outstretched foot.

Te-guruma is a variation on a theme from *sukui-nage*. *Sukui-nage* is when you grab your opponent's legs and pick him/her off the ground (by rolling across your leg whilst turning your body, but not lifting the opponent).

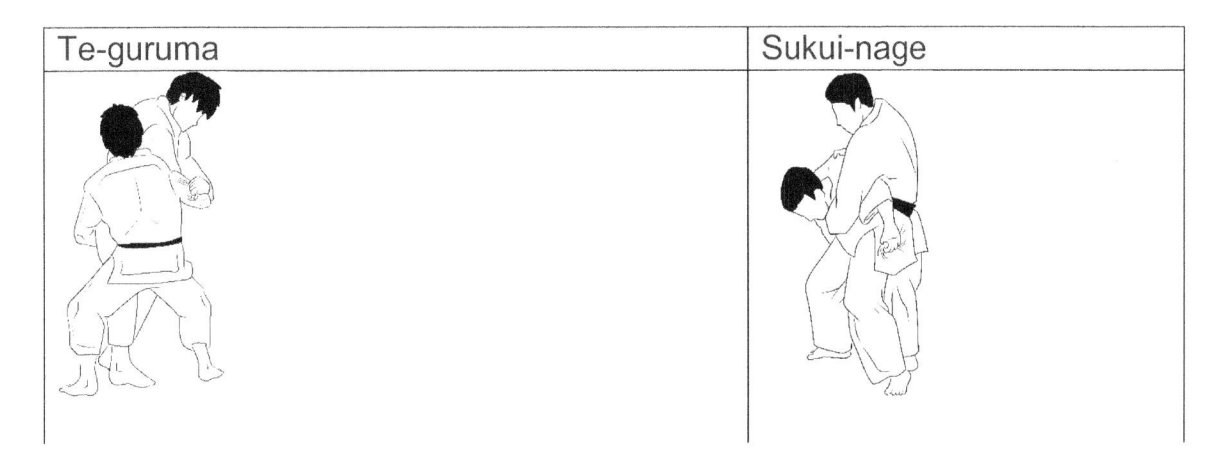

Te-guruma	Sukui-nage

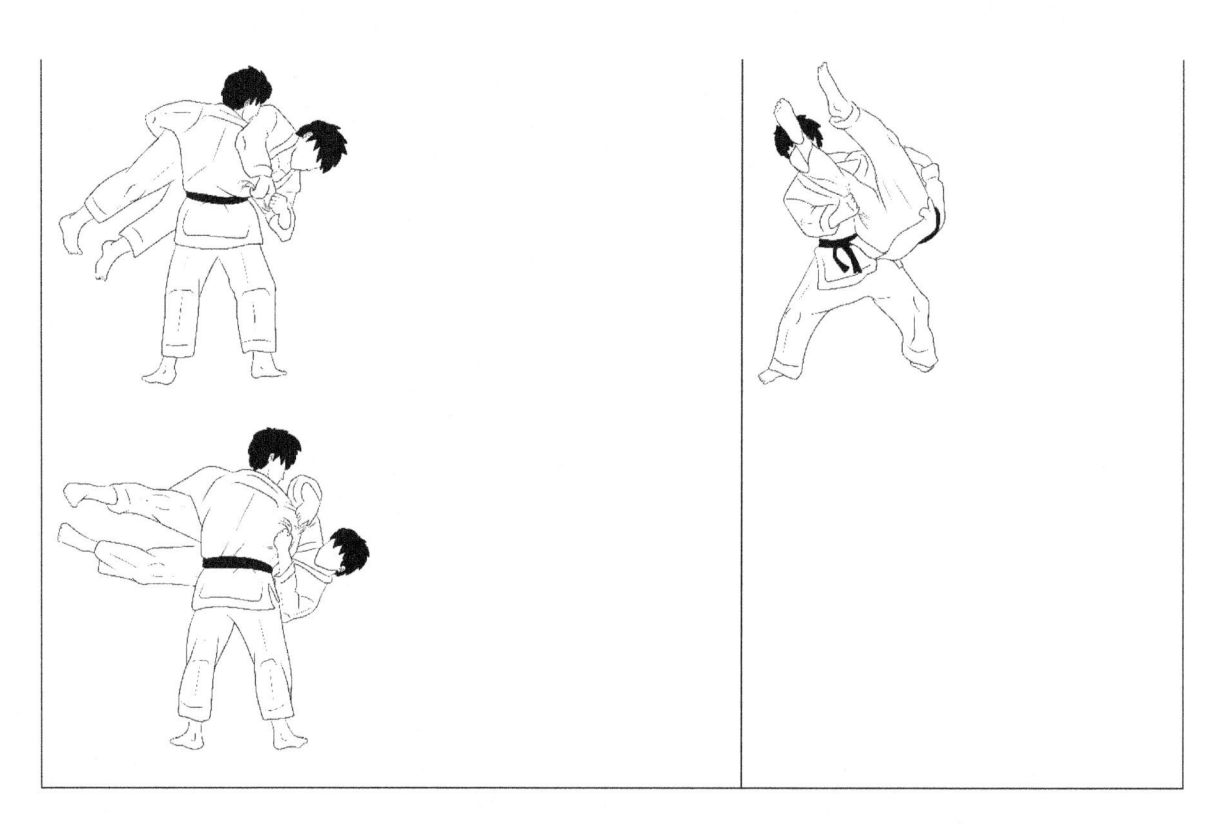

Hybrid Principles

It is possible to vary the combinations of arm and leg positions. For example, start by using inside legs then change to outside legs: *Ko-uchi-gake-maki-komi (can be applied with ippon-seoi-nage hand grips) > ko-soto-maki-komi.*

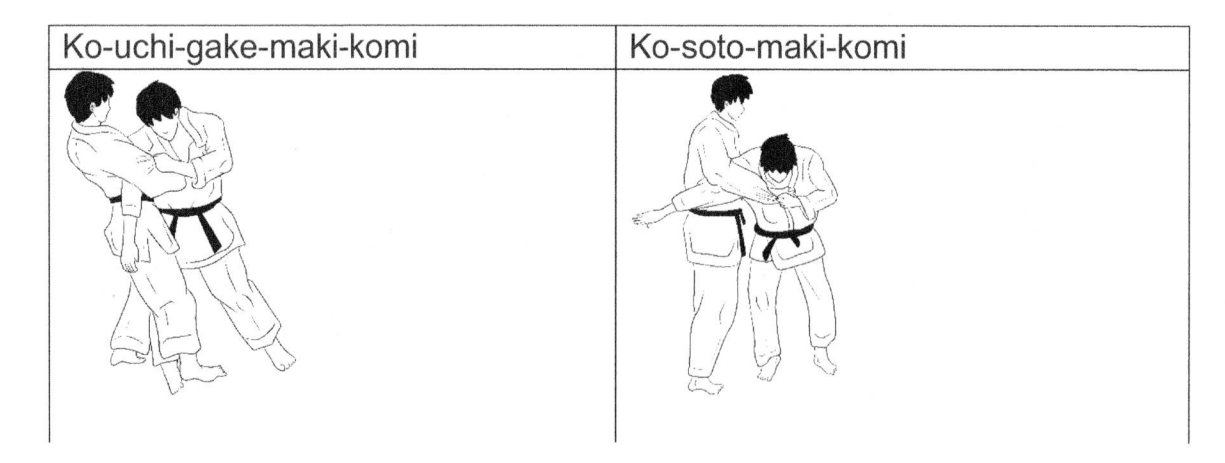

Ko-uchi-gake-maki-komi	Ko-soto-maki-komi

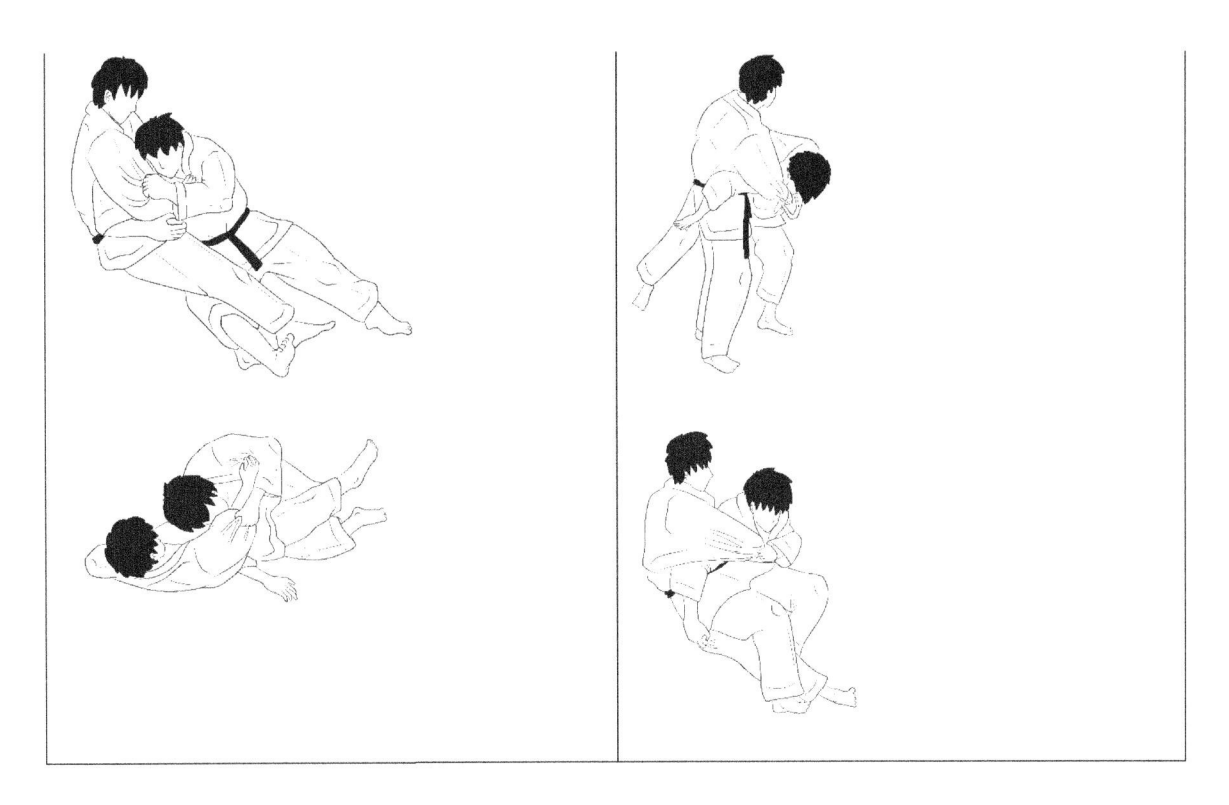

Combine the leg and body grip of *soto-kibisu-gaeshi* with the leg sweep of *o-uchi-gari* to make *soto-ashi-dori-ouchi-gari*.

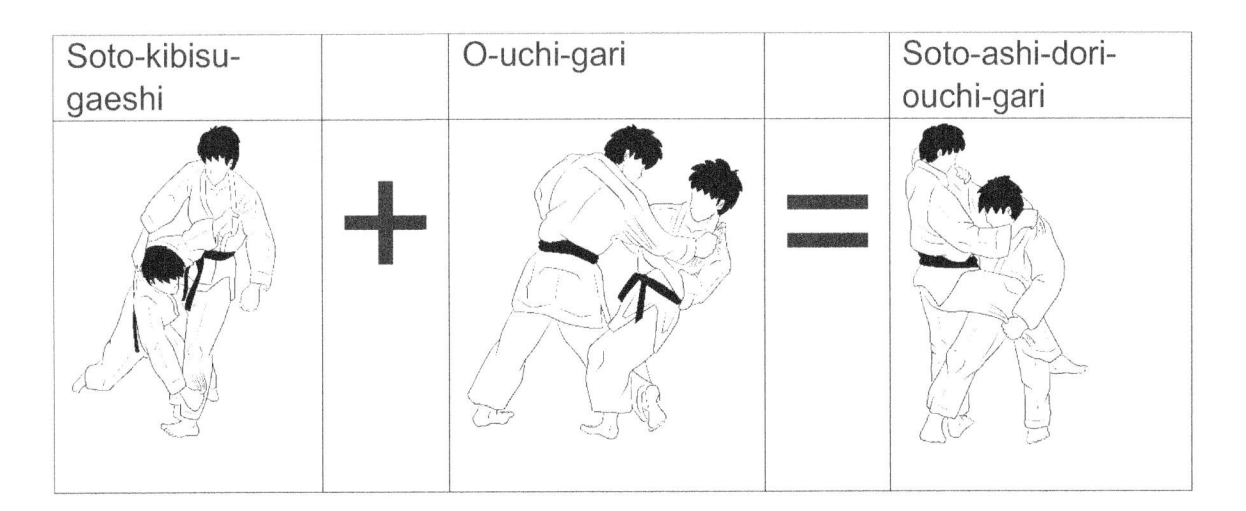

Soto-kibisu-gaeshi		O-uchi-gari		Soto-ashi-dori-ouchi-gari
	+		=	

Combine the forward reaping drive/movement of *soto-kibisu-gaeshi* with leg and body grip plus leg sweep of *kata-uchi-ashi-dori* to make k*ata-hiza-te-ouchi-gake-ashi-dori*.

Soto-kibisu-gaeshi		Kata-uchi-ashi-dori		Kata-hiza-te-ouchi-gake-ashi-dori

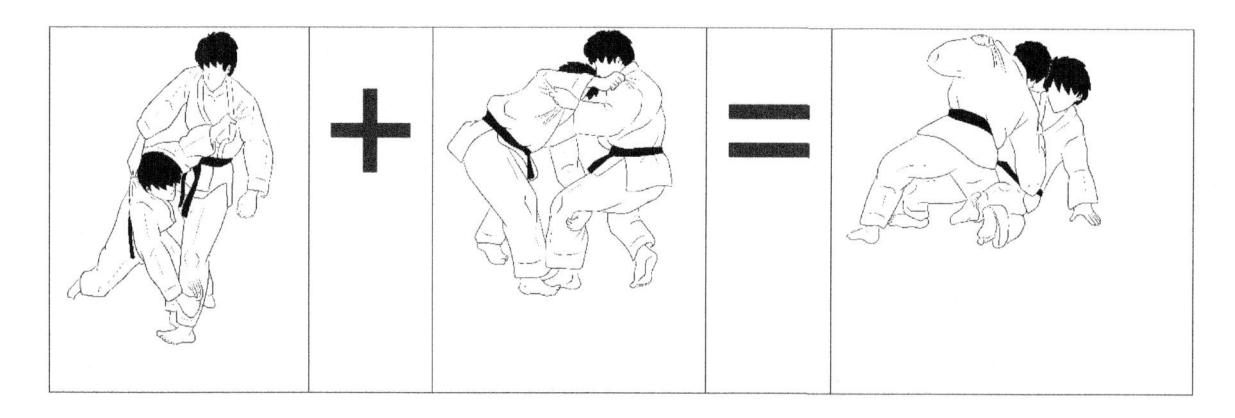

Utsuri-goshi seems impossibly hard until you think of it as combination of *ushiro-goshi* and *o-goshi*. Your opponent tries to throw you with *o-goshi* > Launch them into the air with *ushiro-goshi* > As opponent descends, step in front of them and seize around opponent's waist > *O-goshi*.

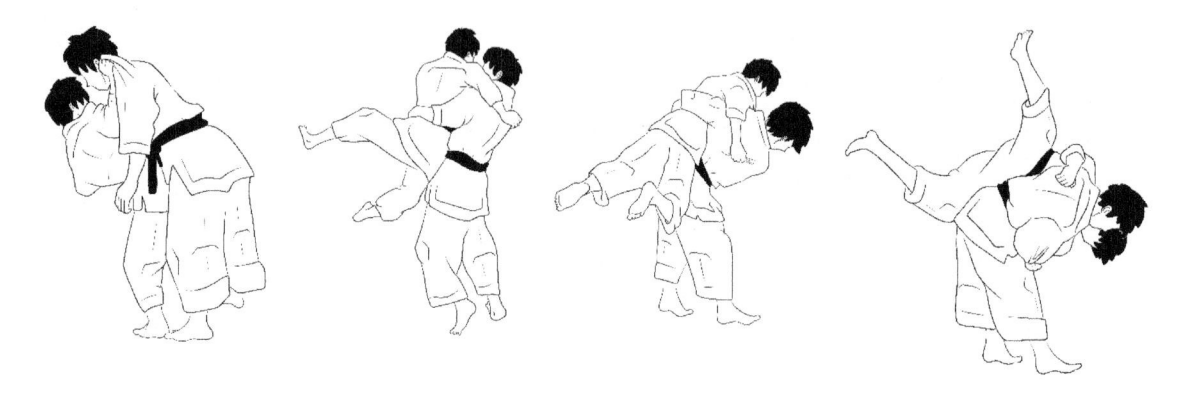

Combine the sleeve and lapel grip of *morote-seoi-nage* with the balancing/supporting leg and leg sweep of *harai-goshi* to make *yama-arashi*.

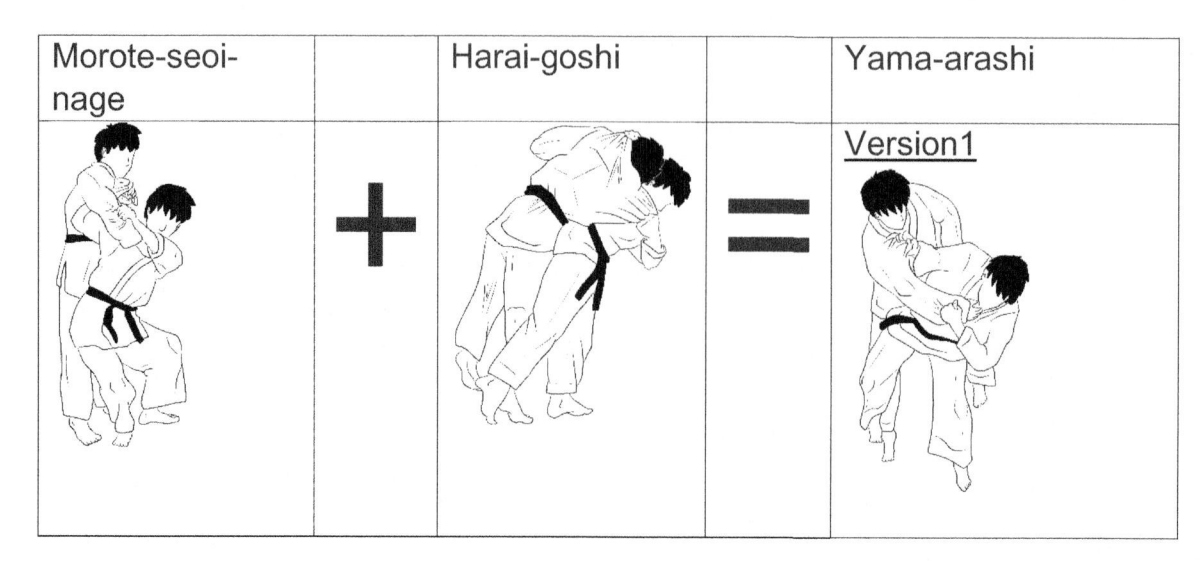

Morote-seoi-nage	Harai-goshi	Yama-arashi
+	=	Version1

Version 2

Modular throw parts of *kani-basami*: Swing leg behind opponent + *hook kick* (reaping leg) + *side break fall* (opposite way to *yoko-wakare*) using 'waterfall' movement principle (as mentioned earlier in the book, under- *More Advanced Principles for Throws and Groundwork*).

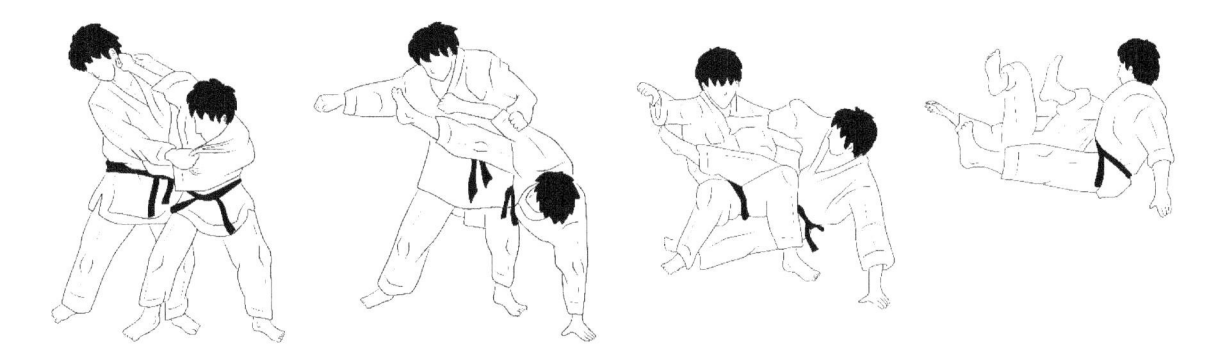

Chapter 6

Groundwork

- Holding Techniques
- Limb Locking Techniques
- Strangling Techniques

Holding Techniques

General Principle

Pin opponent on their back whilst controlling at least one limb.

It is easier to pin your opponent to the mat by controlling their chest/shoulders; this will restrict their movement and ability to break out of a hold.

How to Apply Core Technique

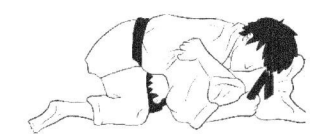

Use your chest to pin down your opponent's chest, and hold him/her in place with your knee(s) and arms.

Variations– "Chest Pin" Techniques

Kami-shiho-gatame	Kuzure-kami-shiho-gatame
Mune-gatame	Kuzure-mune-gatame V1
Kuzure-mune-gatame V2	Gyaku-yoko-shiho-gatame

Yoko-shiho-gatame	Kuzure-yoko-shiho-gatame
Tate-shiho-gatame	Kuzure-tate-shiho-gatame

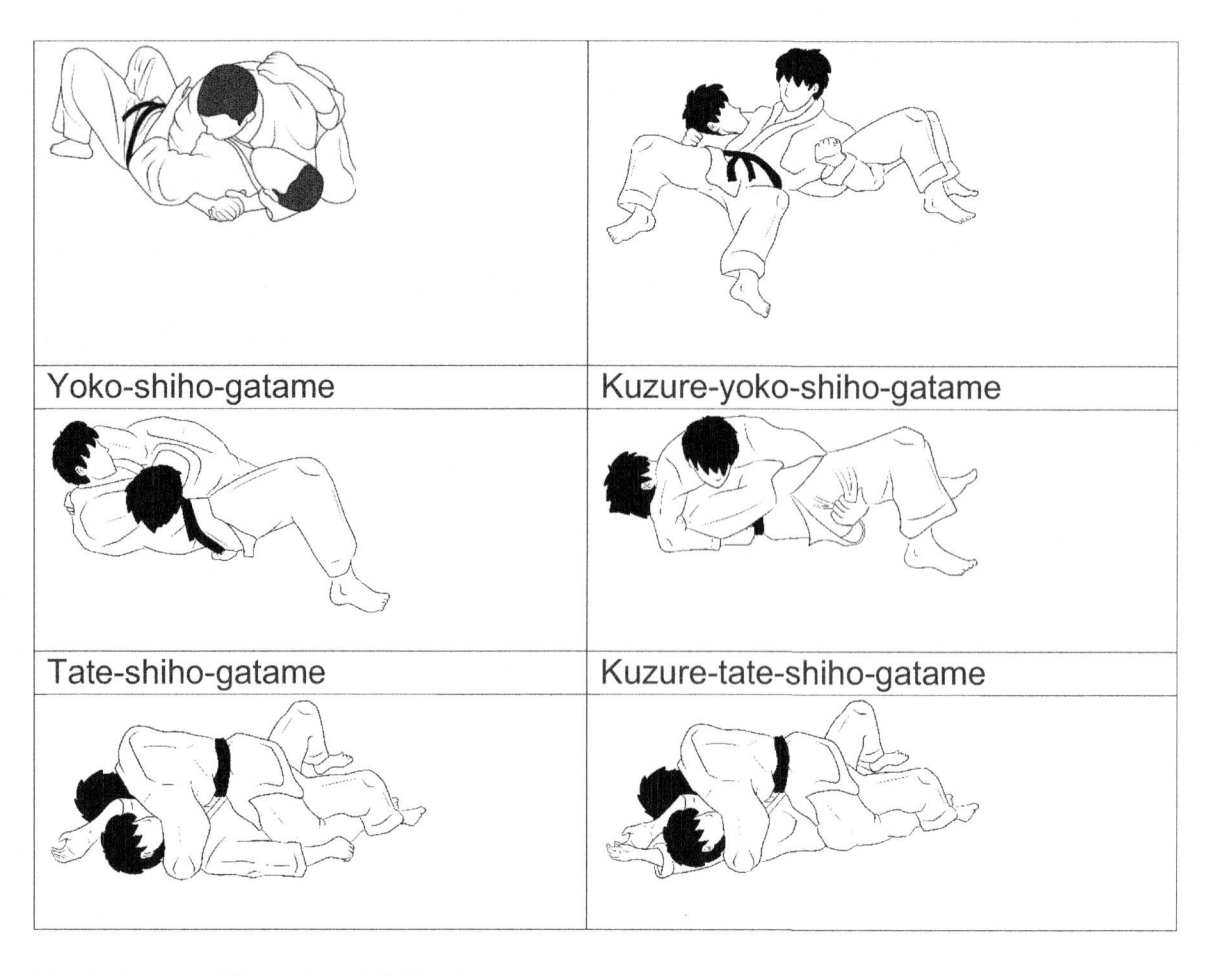

Variations – "Scarf Hold" Techniques

Lie beside your opponent. Clamp one of your opponent's arms into your armpit. Use your other arm to grip opponent. Use grips to wind into opponent's diaphragm and constrict it.

Kesa-gatame	Kuzure-kesa-gatame V1	Kuzure-kesa-gatame V2

Makura-kesa-gatame V1	Makura-kesa-gatame V2	Gyaku-kesa-gatame

Variation – Kata-Gatame

Lie beside your opponent. Clamp one of your opponent's arms between your neck and theirs having reached around their shoulder, then grip own hands. Use grips to wind into opponent's neck/shoulder and constrict them.

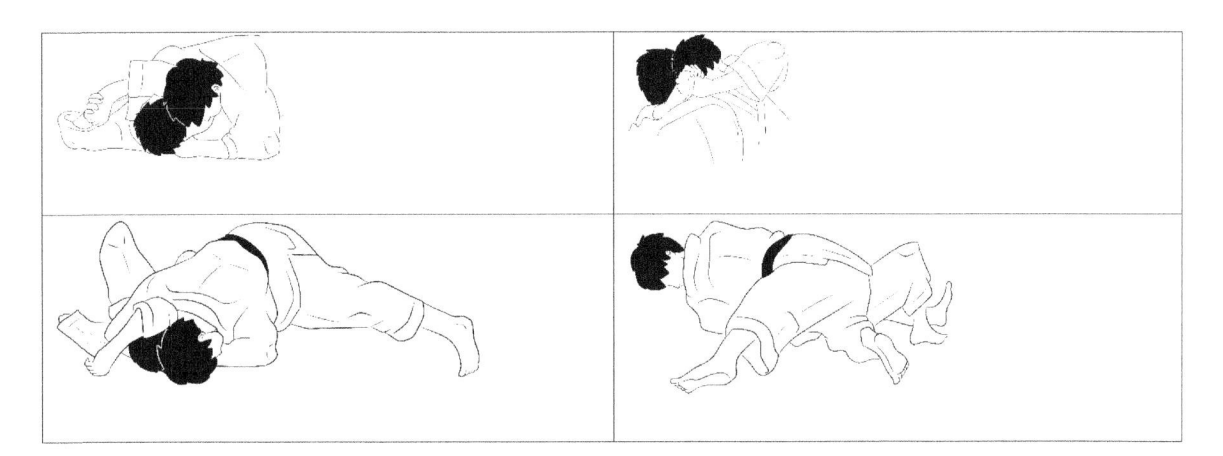

Moving Around the Body

It is possible to move from one hold to another whilst moving:
- Clockwise around opponent's body from (their) right to left.
- Anti-clockwise around opponent's body from (their) left to right.

Diagram showing hold positions around a body:
- Kami-shiho-gatame (top of head)
- Kata-gatame (upper left)
- Gyaku-kesa-gatame (upper right)
- Makura-kesa-gatame V2 (left)
- Mune-gatame (torso)
- Kesa-gatame (left)
- Tate-shiho-gatame (torso)
- Yoko-shiho-gatame (right)

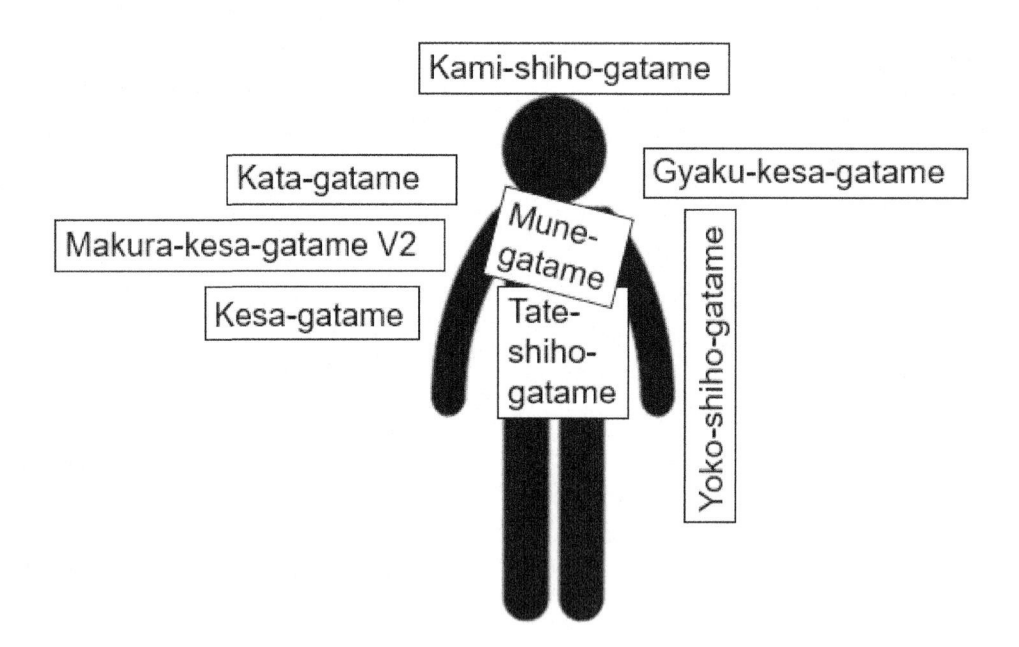

The aim is to hold your opponent down for thirty seconds. If your opponent starts to break out of one hold, move into another.

The *kuzure (broken)* versions of holds can be used instead of the *hon (full/regular)* ones. Or you can use the *kuzure* versions of holds as waypoints when moving between *hon* holds. It is better to establish some degree of control over an opponent through a *kuzure* technique if your opponent has (partially/fully) broken out of a *hon* technique, then work into a position where you can reapply full control with a *hon* technique.

You can move clockwise or anti-clockwise around opponent's body depending on which way they struggle to try and throw you off, and so break the hold.

It is possible to move through all holds in the illustration, or move from one to another without following the exact order.

Some combinations to try:
- As per diagram (*kesa-gatame through to tate-shiho-gatame*).
- *Kesa-gatame > Makura-kesa-gatame V2 > Kata-gatame > Kami-shiho-gatame > Gyaku-kesa-gatame > Yoko-shiho-gatame > Mune-gatame > Tate-shiho-gatame > Kata-gatame >* Return to *Kesa-gatame.*
- *Kami-shiho-gatame > Kuzure-kami-shiho-gatame > Gyaku-kesa-gatame > Kuzure-mune-gatame > Mune-gatame.*

Modular Parts of Holding Techniques

There is less opportunity to mix and match different parts of holding techniques without one technique turning into another. Grips, leg and body positions are predominantly as you see illustrated above in *kesa-gatame*, *kata-gatame*, *kami-shiho-gatame* and *yoko-shiho-gatame*.

There are rare exceptions when you can swap modular parts: Arms, bodies and legs. For example, if you apply *mune-gatame* body and leg parts, with *makura-kesa-gatame* V2 head and shoulder grips; it is possible to switch between *mune-gatame* and *kata-gatame* holds depending on which way your opponent rolls you.

Makura-kesa-gatame V2 > *Mune-gatame* > *Makura-kesa-gatame* V2. Retain *Makura-kesa-gatame* V2 arm hold throughout and simply move your body position.

Limb Locking Techniques

General Principle

The principle behind all (arm) locks is bend a limb in a way it does not want to go.

Leg locks are not generally taught in *judo*. They are used in *ju jitsu* and other martial arts. One reason a ground hold is considered broken in *judo* is when the defender manages to wrap two legs around the attacker's legs. (The attacker being the person applying the ground hold). The hold is considered broken because the defender is in a position to apply a leg lock on the attacker (if these were still widely taught), so the attacker is no longer in control of the defender, and has to try and apply another technique.

The difference between an arm lock and an arm break is speed. They are both the same technique, but the 'break' is applied faster (causing damage to a limb before someone can react or submit).

Strangles and arm locks are traditionally used in groundwork, but can be applied when standing or lying on the ground.

<u>Variations</u>

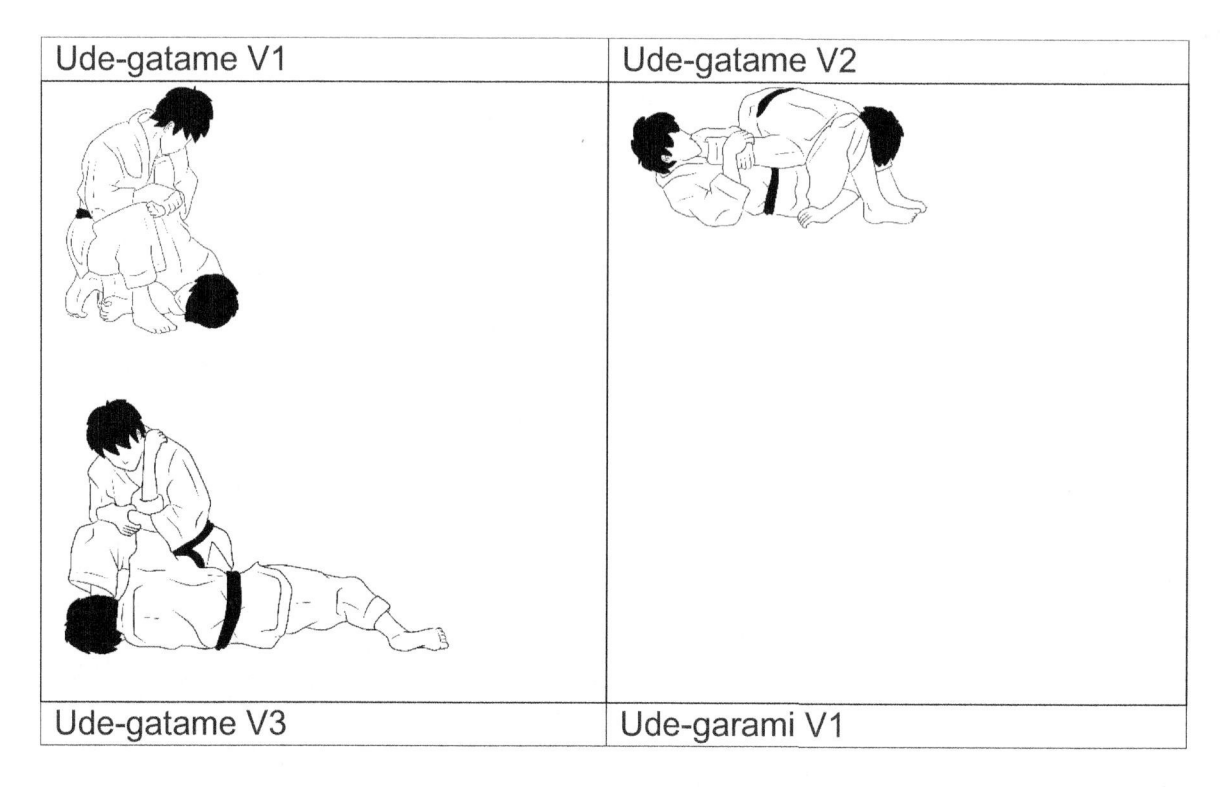

Ude-gatame V1	Ude-gatame V2
Ude-gatame V3	Ude-garami V1

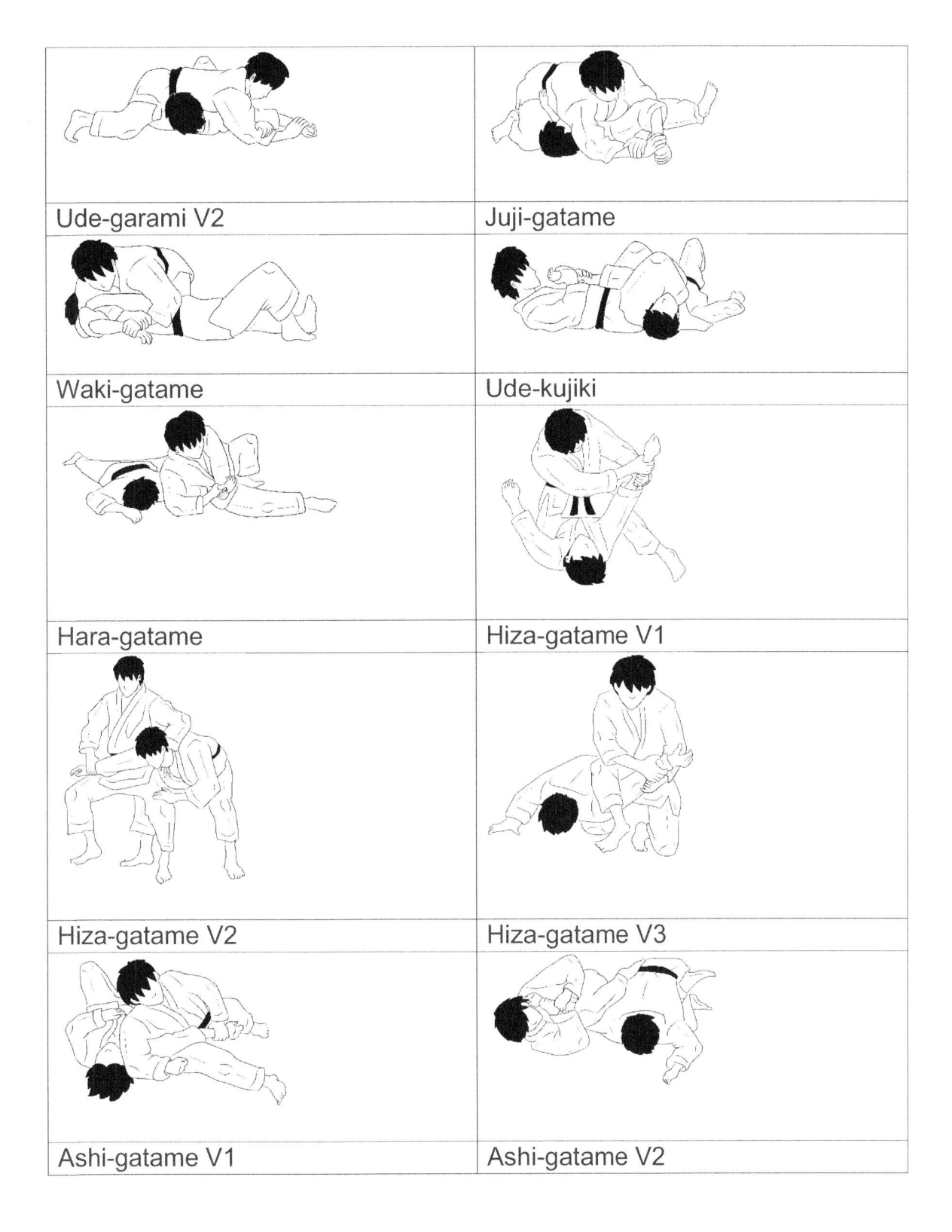

Ude-garami V2	Juji-gatame
Waki-gatame	Ude-kujiki
Hara-gatame	Hiza-gatame V1
Hiza-gatame V2	Hiza-gatame V3
Ashi-gatame V1	Ashi-gatame V2

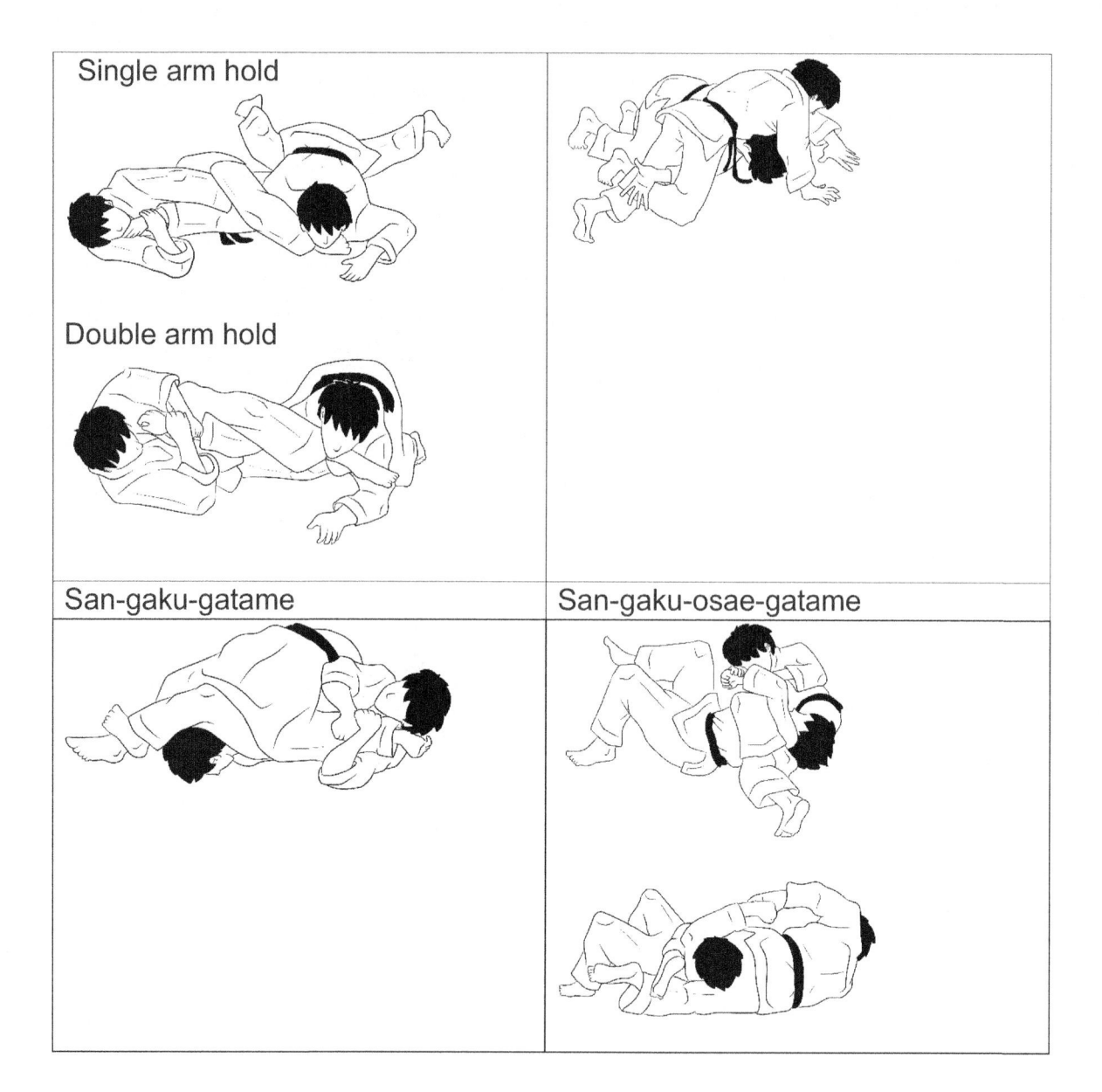

Single arm hold	
Double arm hold	
San-gaku-gatame	San-gaku-osae-gatame

Strangling Techniques

General Principle

Shime-waza is translated as strangling techniques, but in fact covers chokes (the cutting off of air supply through windpipe) and strangles (cutting off blood supply to brain).

As a rule of thumb, you can apply techniques from different positions (standing or in groundwork) as follows:
- Chokes: Throat bar using forearm or *judogi* (*judo* uniform).
- Strangles: Cut off blood supply to side of neck using forearm.

Variations - Chokes

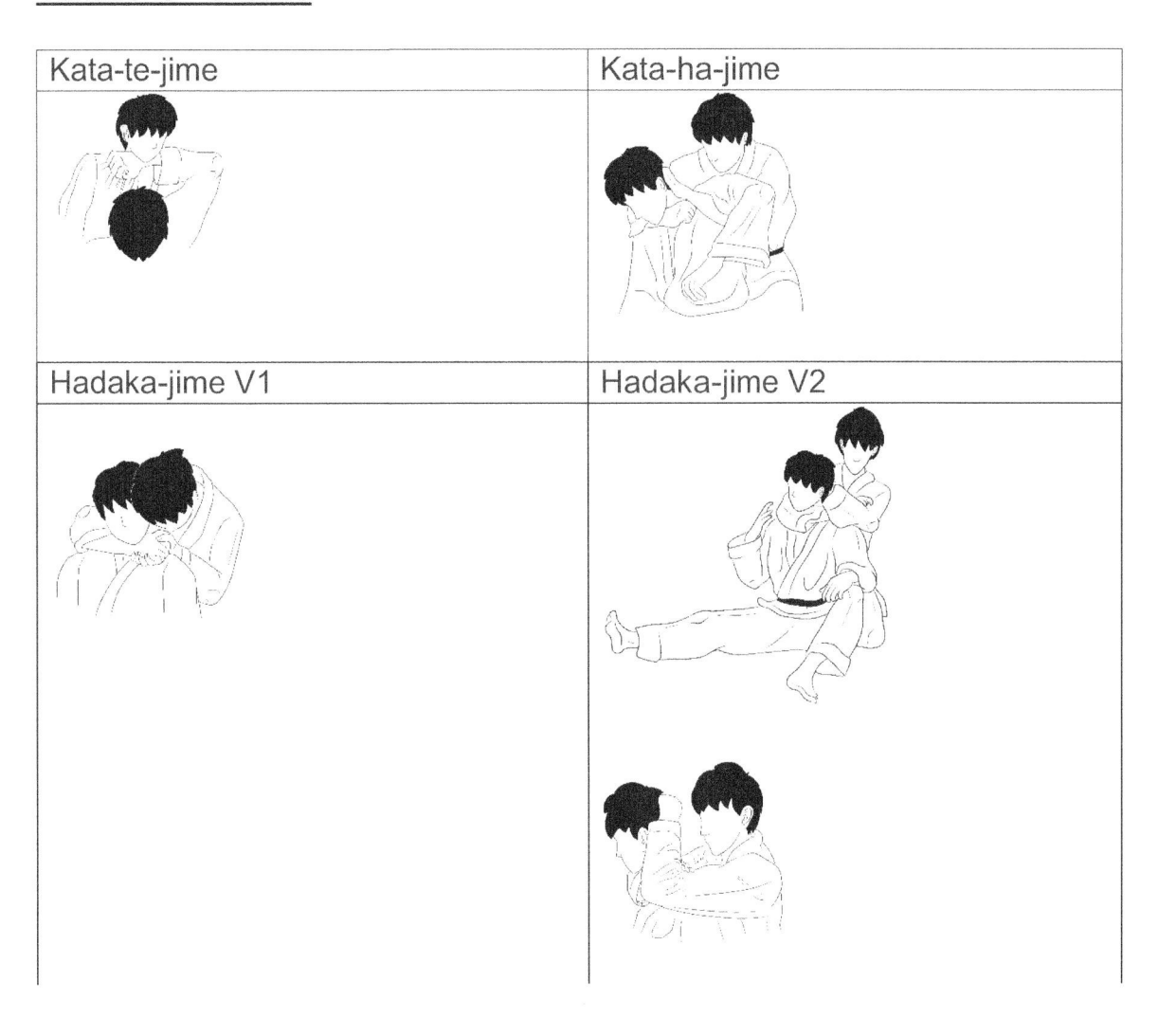

Kata-te-jime	Kata-ha-jime
Hadaka-jime V1	Hadaka-jime V2

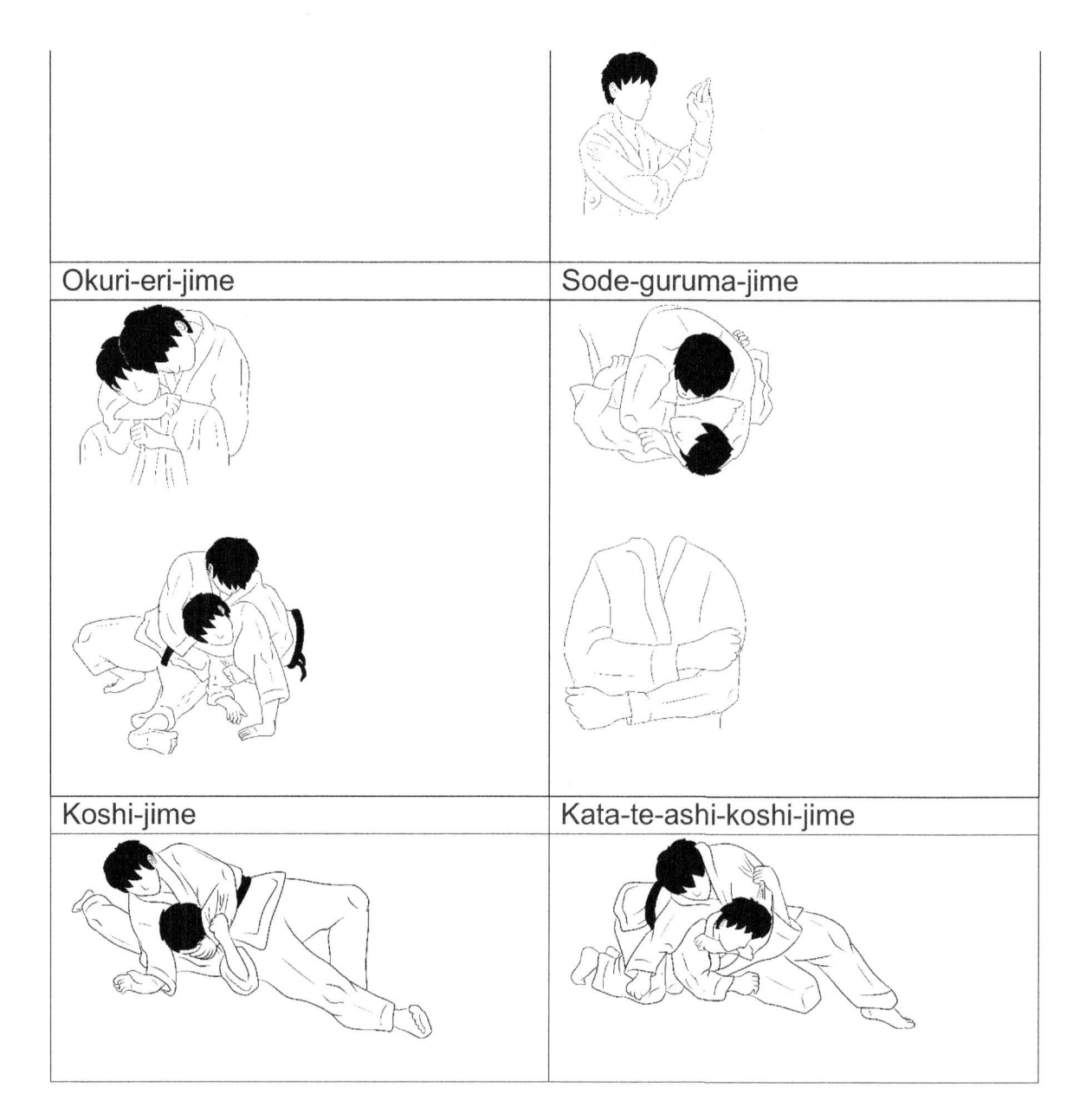

Okuri-eri-jime	Sode-guruma-jime
Koshi-jime	Kata-te-ashi-koshi-jime

Variations - Strangles

The *juji-jimes* are the same strangles in three different positions. You change hand positions and grips. Techniques can be applied face-to-face, on top of, or beneath an opponent.

Gyaku-juji-jime	Kata-juji-jime

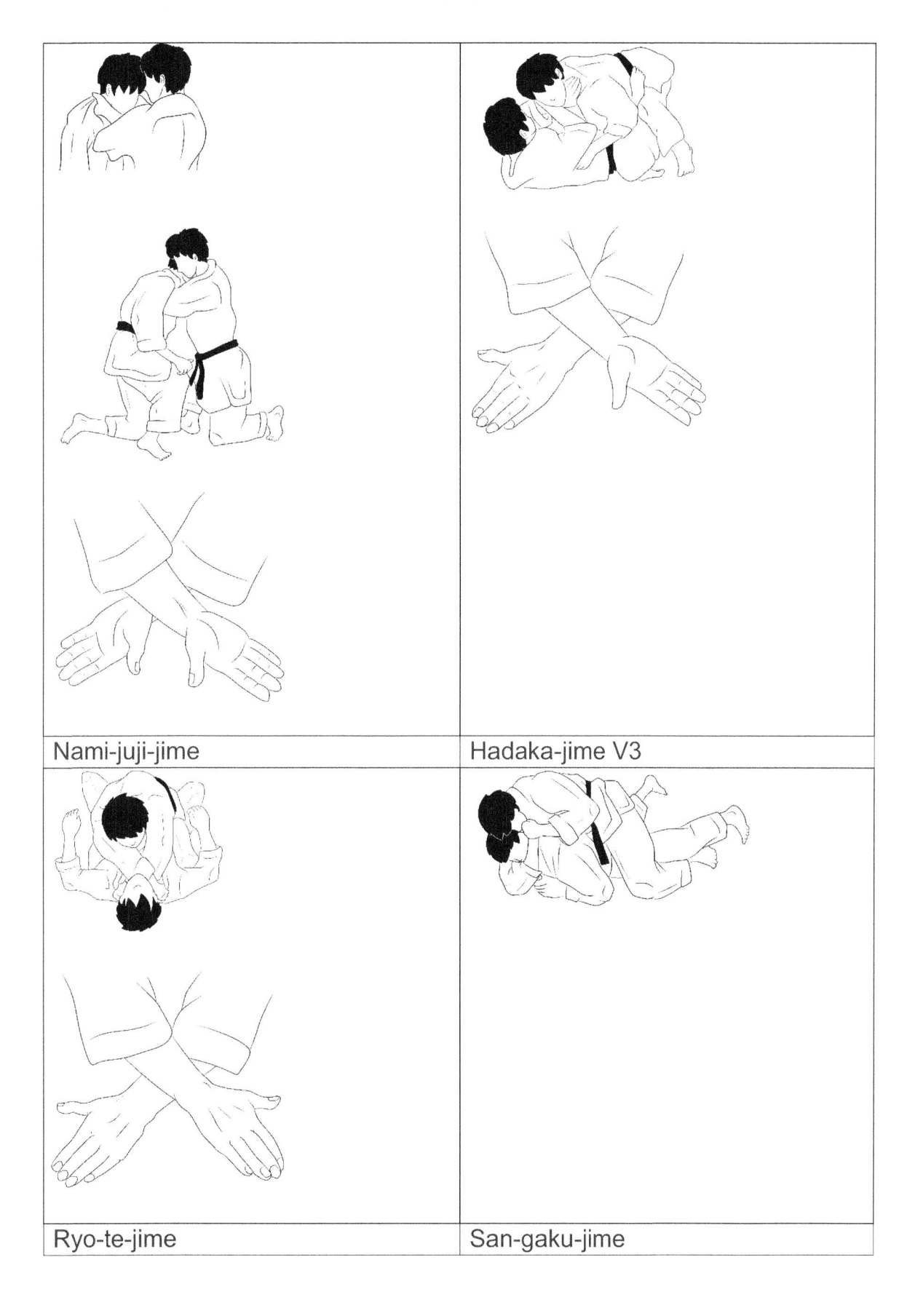

Nami-juji-jime	Hadaka-jime V3
Ryo-te-jime	San-gaku-jime

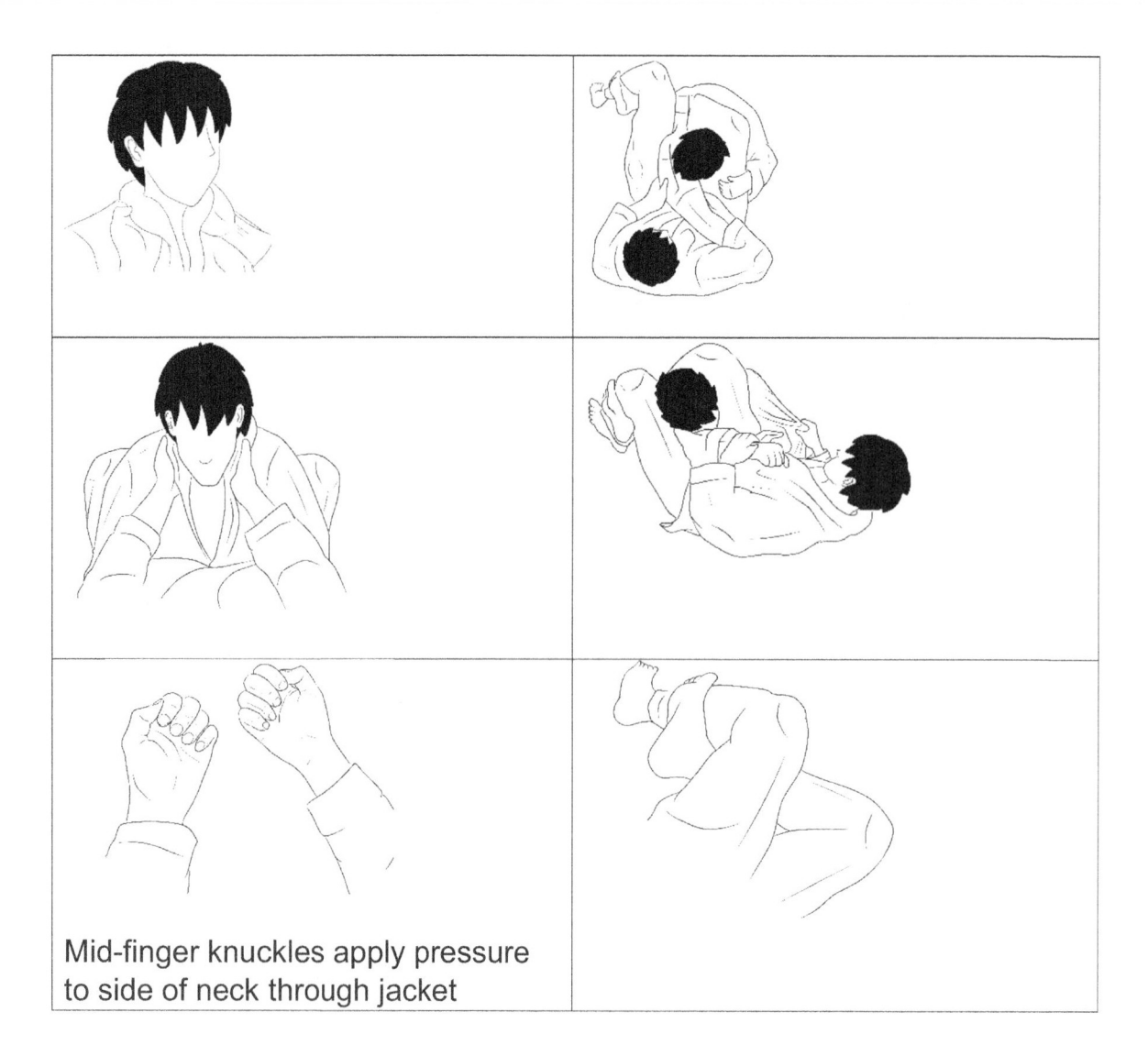

Mid-finger knuckles apply pressure to side of neck through jacket

Postface

Judo Technique List and Glossary

Dedication

Acknowledgements

Judo Technique List

Throwing Techniques

These are known as *tachi-waza* (standing techniques).

Ashi-waza - Foot and Leg Techniques

Ashi-guruma	leg wheel
De-ashi-barai	advancing foot sweep
Harai-tsuri-komi-ashi	sweeping drawing ankle (also known as lifting pulling foot sweep)
Hiza-guruma	knee wheel
Ko-soto-gake	minor outer hook
Ko-soto-gari	minor outer reap
Ko-uchi-gari	minor inner reap
Nidan-ko-soto-gari	furthest leg minor outer reap
O-guruma	major wheel
O-soto-gake	major outer hook
O-soto-gari	major outer reap
O-soto-otoshi	major outer drop
O-uchi-gari	major inner reap
O-soto-guruma	major outer wheel
Okuri-ashi-barai	sliding double foot sweep
Sasae-tsuri-komi-ashi	propping drawing ankle
Soto-ashi-dori-ouchi-gari	outside leg grab (with) major inner sweep
Uchi-mata	inner thigh (throw)

Koshi-waza - Hip Techniques

Hane-goshi	spring hip
Harai-goshi	sweeping loin
Koshi-guruma	hip wheel
O-goshi	major hip
Sode-tsuri-komi-goshi	sleeve lift pull hip (also known as lift sleeve and pull lapel hip throw)
Tsuri-goshi	lifting hip
Tsuri-komi-goshi	drawing hip (lift pull hip)
Uki-goshi	floating hip
Ushiro-goshi	rear hip
Utsuri-goshi	changing hip

Te-waza - Hand Techniques

Ippon-seoi-nage	one-arm shoulder (throw)
Kata-uchi-ashi-dori	single inner (shoulder and) leg grab
Kata-guruma	shoulder wheel
Kata-hiza-te-ouchi-gake-ashi-dori	single knee hand major inside hook (also known as rear leg throw)
Morote-gari	double leg grab/reap
Morote-seoi-nage	two-handed shoulder (throw)
Morote-eri-seoi-nage	two-handed lapel shoulder (throw)
Ryo-hiza-seoi-otoshi	dropping onto two knees shoulder throw
Seoi-otoshi	dropping shoulder (throw)
Soto-kibisu-gaeshi	outer heel trip (leg throw)
Sukui-nage	scooping throw
Sumi-otoshi	corner drop
Tai-otoshi	body drop
Te-guruma	hand wheel
Uchi-kibisu-gaeshi	inner heel trip (leg throw)
Uki-otoshi	floating drop
Yama-arashi	mountain storm

Sutemi-waza - Sacrifice Techniques

Hane-maki-komi	winding spring hip
Hikikomi-gaeshi	rice bale
Kani-basami	scissors throw
Ko-soto-maki-komi	minor outside winding
Ko-uchi-gake-maki-komi	minor inner thigh hook (and one arm) winding (throw); (also known as reclining leg throw)
Soto-maki-komi	outside winding
Sumi-gaeshi	corner throw
Tani-otoshi	valley drop
Tomoe-nage	circle (stomach) throw
Uki-waza	floating throw
Ura-nage	rear throw
Yoko-gake	side hook
Yoko-guruma	side wheel
Yoko-kata-guruma-otoshi	dropping side shoulder wheel
Yoko-otoshi	side drop
Yoko-tomoe-nage	sideways (stomach) circle throw
Yoko-wakare	side separation

Groundwork Techniques

These are known as *ne-waza*.

Kansetsu-waza - Limb Lock Techniques

Ashi-gatame	ankle arm lock
Hara-gatame	stomach arm lock
Hiza-gatame	knee arm lock
Juji-gatame	cross arm lock
San-gaku-gatame	triangular arm lock
San-gaku-osae-gatame	triangular strangle and hold down
Ude-garami	entangled arm lock
Ude-gatame	straight arm lock
Ude-kujiki	smashing arm lock
Waki-gatame	armpit arm lock

Osae-komi-waza - Holding Techniques

Gyaku-kesa-gatame	reverse scarf hold
Gyaku-yoko-shiho-gatame	reverse side four quarters hold
Kami-shiho-gatame	upper four quarters hold
Kata-gatame	shoulder hold
Kesa-gatame	scarf hold
Kuzure-kami-shiho-gatame	broken upper four quarters hold
Kuzure-kesa-gatame	broken scarf hold
Kuzure-mune-gatame	broken chest (crushing) hold
Kuzure-tate-shiho-gatame	broken straddling four quarters hold
Kuzure-yoko-shiho-gatame	broken side four quarters hold
Makura-kesa-gatame	pillow scarf hold
Mune-gatame	chest (crushing) hold
Tate-shiho-gatame	straddling four quarters hold
Yoko-shiho-gatame	side four quarters hold

Shime-waza - Strangling Techniques

Gyaku-juji-jime	reverse cross strangle
Hadaka-jime	naked strangle/choke
Kata-ha-jime	single collar strangle
Kata-juji-jime	half cross strangle
Kata-te-ashi-koshi-jime	single hand leg hip strangle/choke
Kata-te-jime	strangle with one hand (also known as single arm throat bar)

Koshi-jime	hip strangle/choke
Nami-juji-jime	normal cross strangle
Okuri-eri-jime	sliding collar strangle/choke
Ryo-te-jime	double hand strangle
San-gaku-jime	triangular strangle
Sode-guruma-jime	sleeve wheel strangle

Glossary of Terms

There are many terms you can learn in *judo*. Below are the ones I use in my book.

Judogi	*judo* uniform
Hon	full/regular/standard (hold)
Judoka	judo practitioner (someone who does judo)
Kata	a formal system of pre-arranged/stylised movements
Kodomo-no-kata	forms for children
Kuzure	broken (hold), can also apply to a variation (i.e. anything that is not the 'standard' technique)
Ma-sutemi-waza	back sacrifice throws
Ne-waza	groundwork techniques
Nage-waza	throwing techniques
Opponent	the person in front of you when using techniques. Can be a training partner when practising, someone you are trying to score points off in a competition or someone you are fighting in self-defence.
Randori	free practice
Tai-sabaki	body movement
Yoko-sutemi-waza	side sacrifice throws

Dedication

To my instructors in various martial arts over the years. With particular thanks to the following teachers:

Richard Drage
Ickleton Judo Club
For teaching me to be a better student, and to see the patterns in martial arts

Thank you for being a sensei, not just in *judo*, but also in how to approach life. The way you taught me over many years has influenced how I teach others at work and in my other hobbies

Kevin Parker
Hatfield Academy of Martial Arts
Thank you for teaching me and giving me the confidence to try something new

Peter Monkman
Hatfield Academy of Martial Arts
For getting me into martial arts, which is now a long-term passion

Acknowledgements

Susanna West Yates
As editor in chief – thank you for all your help and support.

Proof Readers
Thank you for all your proof reading: Andrew, Eve, Geoff, Mike and Tris.

Illustrators
'jprs_n', 'ramanafis' and special thanks in particular to 'Ankaramedia' as lead illustrator

Thank you for your patience and attention to detail when illustrating the figures in this book.

About the Author

James Goddard

James has an extensive interest in martial arts, which he has been practising for a number of years. He has experience of six martial arts spread over nine styles.

James noticed there were patterns and crossovers in principles of movement in martial arts. This is what inspired him to write this book.

James has also been dancing Ballroom and Latin for many years.

James often jokes he uses more *judo* on the dance floor than on the *judo* mat…

If you liked this book, please look out for the *Goddard Method of Ballroom and Latin Dancing*. This will explain how to do Ballroom and Latin in a similar style to the way James approached *judo* in this book.

James has also published a fiction book called *Ellie's Magical Cat*.

You can find out details about, and specials offers for, James' books on https://jamesgoddarddancing.wordpress.com

Printed in Great Britain
by Amazon